HORMONAL REGULATION
OF FARM ANIMAL GROWTH

Hormonal Regulation of Farm Animal Growth

K.L. Hossner

Department of Animal Sciences
Colorado State University
Fort Collins, Colorado
USA

CABI Publishing

CABI Publishing is a division of CAB International

CABI Publishing
CAB International
Wallingford
Oxfordshire OX10 8DE
UK

CABI Publishing
875 Massachusetts Avenue
7th Floor
Cambridge, MA 02139
USA

Tel: +44 (0)1491 832111
Fax: +44 (0)1491 833508
E-mail: cabi@cabi.org
Website: www.cabi-publishing.org

Tel: +1 617 395 4056
Fax: +1 617 354 6875
E-mail: cabi-nao@cabi.org

A catalogue record for this book is available from the British Library, London, UK.

Library of Congress Cataloging-in-Publication Data

Hossner, K. L. (Kim L.)
    Hormonal regulation of farm animal growth / K.L. Hossner.
        p. cm.
    Includes bibliographical references and index.
    ISBN-10: 0-85199-080-0 (alk. paper)
    ISBN-13: 978-0-85199-080-4 (alk. paper)
1. Livestock--Growth--Regulation. 2. Hormones. 3. Growth regulators. I. Title.

SF768.H67 2005
636.08'52--dc22   2005005787

ISBN 0 85199 080 0

Typeset by SPI Publisher Services, Pondicherry, India
Printed and bound in the UK by Cromwell Press, Trowbridge

Contents

1 Whole Animal Growth

The primary focus of this book is to examine the regulation of farm animal growth by hormones and growth factors, primarily at the cell and molecular level. As such, most of this book will be devoted to the study of developmental, cellular and molecular mechanisms that are involved with the regulation of cell and tissue growth. This chapter is designed to provide a cursory outline of some of the most basic aspects of whole animal growth. I hope that this chapter will inform readers of the processes involved with animal growth and expose them to some of the factors that influence growth and its measurement at the organismal level.

Measuring Animal Growth

The study of animal growth can be undertaken at several levels, ranging from the cellular and molecular to whole animal studies. At the cellular level, growth may be quantitated by measuring the increase in cell size and cell number. This can be done directly by counting numbers of cells or by measuring changes in their size using a microscope. We can also measure cell number or mass indirectly, using chemical analysis. As the amount of DNA in a cell is constant, quantitation of DNA concentration per unit mass can be used as an accurate reflection of cell numbers. In addition, the use of the other primary cell macromolecules, RNA and protein, can be measured as a reflection of cell, tissue or organ mass. These are somewhat less accurate than using DNA measurements, as the amount of protein and RNA may change as a result of experimental treatment. At the organ level, changes in organ mass or function can be quantitated during different developmental stages or in response to experimental treatments. At the whole animal level, growth parameters can be quantitated during different portions of the life cycle. The study of growth can focus on changes that occur during embryonic and fetal growth, or during the postnatal period that occurs immediately after parturition. Some studies are focused on pre-pubertal growth, the time between birth and puberty. Of interest in animal husbandry is the 'fattening' phase of adult animal growth, when farm animals have essentially ended their linear growth but continue to accumulate fat, altering their body composition and the characteristic flavour of the meat derived from these animals.

At the cell level, growth can occur in two ways. Cells can replicate via the process of mitosis to increase overall mass by increasing cell numbers. This process of cell replication is called hyperplasia. The second way in which cells can grow is to increase in size or volume. This process is known as hypertrophy. During the formation of organs during embryogenesis and in cells grown in tissue culture, cells initially increase their numbers by mitotic replication, cease replication and then grow by expanding in size. The growth in size or volume of cells is accompanied by protein synthesis, and in the case of adipocytes, by accumulation of large amounts of lipid. Cellular hypertrophy is especially prominent during the development of the large cells characteristic of mature adipose tissue and skeletal muscle. This postmitotic alteration in cell size and shape is accompanied by qualitative alterations in gene expression. As a result, cells change from relatively simple, proliferating cells into differentiated cells that assume specialized functions associated with the mature organ. For example, the development of specialized intracellular structures such as contractile fibres in muscle or intracellular accumulation of large amounts of lipid that serves as energy storage depots in adipocytes.

Animal growth is a quantitative factor that can be measured objectively. In the living animal, as bones lengthen during linear growth, changes in body weight, height or length accompany growth. In addition, qualitative changes occur in body proportions and functions, which accompany maturation and the increase in body size. The study of the changes in body proportions during growth is called allometry. At the whole animal level, growth is measured by an increase in length of bony appendages (height or length), or the enhanced growth of muscles and organs. Quantitative increase in muscle mass is important for animal producers and ultimately, consumers. The quality of muscle growth is also of importance for the production of meat for consumption and the ratio of intramuscular fat to muscle is an important measure of meat quality.

The simplest and most commonly used method to measure whole animal growth is to simply measure body weight. But when doing this, one must be aware that simple body weights may reflect water accumulation, gut fill, fat deposition, as well as wet hide weight and faecal contamination, not necessarily true growth. Thus, it is important to obtain body weight of different animals under identical conditions of husbandry, so that effects of feeding and watering, as well as transportation, are eliminated. Animals, which are transported over long distances, in some cases for many days, arrive at their destinations dehydrated and underfed. Rapid rehydration by excess water consumption leads to falsely high body weights. Body weights for cattle obtained after 24 h without feed, but with access to water, provide a 'shrunk body weight', which is highly correlated with empty body weight, i.e. the weight of the body minus the gut contents.

Embryonic and Fetal Growth

Growth is composed of two basic components that occur sequentially, but overlap over time. As discussed earlier, true growth consists of an increase in mass, length and height of an animal. At the same time there is a change in body form or proportions. This is due to the differential growth of tissues and is most evident in fetal development. As shown in Fig. 1.1, the changes in body proportions that accompany growth from the human fetus to the adult change dramatically. During development, the head and brain develop first and in the early fetus, the head occupies one-half of the body length, while in the adult, it accounts for about one-eighth of the body length. In contrast, the hind limbs develop later, occupying only an one-eighth of the body length in the fetus, but roughly one-half in the adult. Changes in body proportions or form also play a role in the ultimate body shape of farm animals and form the criteria for judging animals in the show ring and determining fat content in the feedlot. In mature humans this is best seen in sedentary individuals who, as a result of differential fat deposition, adopt an apple or pear-shaped body form over time. Development of optimal proportions of the major tissues involved with animal production, muscle, bone and fat, are essential to produce an animal which is economically efficient to manage and produces a relatively large proportion of meat which is acceptable to the consumer. A high amount of muscle with a minimum amount of bone and fat is an ideal condition for meat animals. The most efficient animals are those that rapidly gain weight and reach a mature body size with less body fat. Cattle being fed during the feedlot phase of production have essentially ceased linear growth and now accumulate subcutaneous fat and demonstrate the altered proportions of a relatively sedentary animal.

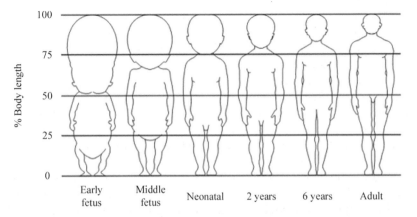

Fig. 1.1. Changes in body proportions during development. Adapted from Stratz (1909).

During embryonic growth, tissues grow sequentially (Fig. 1.2), proceeding from anterior to posterior during development. In early embryos the components of the central nervous system (CNS), the brain and spinal cord, develop first. Bone formation follows shortly thereafter and overlaps CNS development. The bones form the scaffolding around which muscle cells form and attach during fetal development. Adipose tissue is the last tissue to develop. Adipose tissue is formed primarily during postnatal development, although some adipose tissue primordia are formed during embryogenesis in many species. Adipose tissue is primarily a tissue of maturity, which is used to store excess energy in the form of fat, or triglycerides. This occurs in the postnatal period when nutritional energy is abundant and is in excess of the body's requirements for energy utilization.

Growth Curves

Whole animal growth can be described in several ways using different types of growth curves (Fig. 1.3). Probably the most common way of describing growth is to simply plot height or weight of the animal vs time (Fig. 1.3A). This results in a sigmoidal curve that is characteristic of the growth of many living organisms, including animals and their organs and plants and their components. Bacterial colonies and animal cells grown *in vitro* also follow sigmoidal growth curves. The sigmoidal growth curve is characterized by an

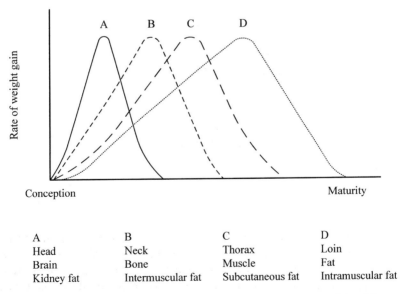

A	B	C	D
Head	Neck	Thorax	Loin
Brain	Bone	Muscle	Fat
Kidney fat	Intermuscular fat	Subcutaneous fat	Intramuscular fat

Fig. 1.2. Growth rates of body regions and tissues during development. Adapted from Hammond (1955).

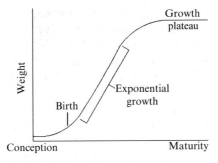

(A) Sigmoidal growth curve

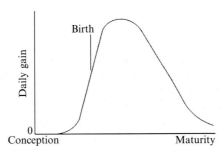

(B) Daily gain growth curve

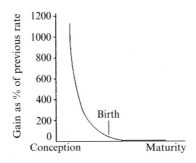

(C) Percent increment growth curve

Fig. 1.3. Types of growth curves.

initial exponential growth phase, when growth is very rapid and the slope of the curve is maximal. The exponential phase is followed by an inflection point when the shape of the curve changes from the very rapid growth of the young organism to a more moderate, slower growth rate. Finally, the growth rate reaches the growth plateau, when growth is very slow and essentially ceases.

Another type of growth curve is derived by plotting the average daily weight gain against the age of animal (Fig. 1.3B). This curve emphasizes the rapid growth rates seen during the postnatal period, culminating in the high growth rate during the time of maturation, followed by a slow decline in growth rate until mature size is reached. Fig. 1.3C shows the per cent increment growth curve. In this curve, the percentage increase in body weight is compared to the previous weight. This curve emphasizes the extremely rapid growth of the early fetus – over a 1000% rate – which rapidly declines in the postnatal animal.

Genetics, Nutrition and Environmental Effects on Whole Animal Growth

The most important of the factors that control whole animal growth are the animal's genetic background, its nutritional intake and the environment that the animal is exposed to. These factors have provided the fundamental basis for the traditional control and manipulation of animal growth throughout the history of animal agriculture. They are the most obvious and visible variables that affect the growth of all organisms, including humans, which can be controlled to optimize the production of farm animals. Optimal growth, production and health of animals depend upon an animal with good genetic qualities that are reflected with the phenotype of the animal. Likewise, animals must be provided with adequate nutritional resources in order to survive and produce a product of quality. Animals maintained in a sheltered environment that is protected from extreme temperature and climatic fluctuations will perform better than those that are not. As a major proportion of the animal sciences curriculum focuses on these factors, these topics will be discussed only briefly. One should keep in mind that hormones of the endocrine system are influenced by all of these factors: genetics, nutrition and environmental stresses. As a rule, these parameters are under rigid experimental control when endocrine studies are carried out.

Genetics

The genetic background of an animal provides the fundamental capacity for rapid growth, body composition and adult size. The genetic background of an animal encompasses all heritable traits. These include such things as coat colour and density, bone structure, growth rates, muscling and fat deposition. While some of these characteristics are simple, single gene-mediated, dominant or recessive traits, most inherited traits of interest to animal producers are the result of the effects of multiple genes working cooperatively. These traits, called quantitative traits, are the cumulative result of tens or hundreds of genes working together. The genetic background of an animal provides the basic potential for ultimate growth rate and mature size (height and weight).

Characteristics of animal growth are heritable and contribute to the large variation seen in animal body sizes and growth rates. One only has to look at the wide variation in the shape and size of dogs to see the effects of genetics and genetic selection, on morphology and body size. Dog breeds range in size from a few ounces in Mexican Chihuahuas to a few hundred pounds in Saint Bernards. The long-legged, lean body form of racing breeds such as the greyhounds and whippets is in stark contrast to the short, pug-faced English bulldogs or the small, short-legged Dachshunds. The heritability of growth characteristics accounts for 25% to 30% of the variation in growth. Some of the heritable traits can be attributed to major gene effects and single genes have been implicated in several instances in which growth or body composition are altered. The double-muscling phenotype of Belgian blue and Piedmontese cattle that actually results from muscle hypertrophy is due to a mutation of the myostatin gene. The naturally occurring myostatin gene acts to limit muscle growth and cattle inheriting the mutant inactive form undergo significant muscle hypertrophy associated with the double-muscling phenotype. Callipyge sheep are also characterized by muscle hypertrophy, but in this case, hypertrophy is localized to the hind limbs and sheep with this phenotype have large hindquarters (callipyge means 'beautiful buttocks' in Greek). This distinct alteration of morphology is due to a single non-recessive gene inherited from the sire.

In contrast, most complex phenotypic traits, such as the graded, continuous variation seen in animal body size, growth rates and body composition result from the cooperative effects of many genes, each with a variable contribution to a specific complex phenotypic trait. These multigene effects are called quantitative traits and are the primary focus of breeding and selection in animal agriculture. In sheep and cattle, selection has centred on body weight at a specific age, either weaning weight in sheep or weaning, yearling or 18 months weights in cattle. Rate of growth, measured as average daily gain (ADG), is often used as a selection criterion in farm animals. In contrast to cattle and sheep, pigs have a relatively short generation time and produce multiple offspring, making them more amenable to selection studies. Selection for higher growth rates in swine over ten generations leads to rapid improvements in production characteristics. Growth rates, measured as ADG, can be increased by almost 50%, while feed intake is increased by about 35% and efficiency of feed utilization increased by about 13%.

The advent of molecular biological methods has allowed the use of molecular genetic markers as selection criteria in farm animals. Two general types of genetic markers are used for improvement of production characteristics, single locus markers and multiple locus markers. Single locus markers represent a single gene of particular significance, one that is associated with major production traits, such as the genes for the hormones leptin, growth hormone (GH) or insulin-like growth hormone-I (IGF-I). These hormones are associated with body composition, growth rates and birth and weaning weights. As such, they exert effects on multiple organ systems including bone, muscle and fat as well as the overall energy metabolism and nutrient partitioning in the body. At the molecular level, genes for single hormones exist as molecular alleles that have variable overall lengths, as measured in the number of bases of DNA that comprise a specific gene. These molecular alleles may confer tissue specificity of gene expression or may result in a gene product that has enhanced biological activity. In addition, alterations in the sizes or numbers of gene regulatory elements associated with specific alleles may increase or decrease the response of a gene to factors that regulate the activity of a certain gene. These single gene alleles may be studied at the molecular level using restriction fragment length polymorphism (RFLP). These fragments of DNA from specific genes are generated using restriction endonucleases, which cut the gene at specific sites, or by PCR amplification of specific gene sites. This generates a set of two or three RFLP fragments of the gene, which represent the molecular alleles. The RFLPs can then be used as selection markers. The use of RFLPs as genetic markers provides limited information from only a single gene and the use of multiple single gene markers in a single individual or breed is more likely to provide useful selection information. To date, the use of single gene markers to improve production characteristics has not proven to be very useful for selection studies.

As hormones are present in the circulation, another approach has been to use genetic selection based on systemic hormone levels, with the assumption that gene activity is reflected by concentrations of hormones in the bloodstream and that a single hormone can effectively alter growth, growth rates and metabolism. The utilization of hormones as genetic markers must be done with the knowledge that hormone concentrations are influenced by many variables other than genetics, including developmental stage, breed, nutrition, time of day or year and so on. The earliest hormones used for this approach included insulin and thyroid hormones, which are related to growth and differentiation. Due to the unwanted metabolic side effects of these hormones (e.g. abnormal lipid, carbohydrate and protein metabolism), their use as selection tools has not been fruitful. Another hormone used for this type of analysis was GH, which is associated with growth rate and lean tissue growth. This use of GH in selection studies (and all studies) is complicated by the fluctuations in serum GH concentrations seen on a minute-to-minute basis. To accurately measure GH, blood samples must be drawn at 10 to 15 min intervals for a 6 to 8 h period. As GH concentrations are also affected by stress and nutrient intake, these variables must also be carefully controlled. Results of selection based on GH concentrations have been inconsistent and animals selected for increased levels result in either fat deposition or leaner phenotypes. IGF-I is a hormone that mediates the effects of GH. Unlike GH, IGF-I serum concentrations are constant and single blood samples are adequate to establish circulating concentrations. Concentrations of IGF-I are correlated with body weight and growth rate in sheep, cattle, pigs and chickens. Selection based on IGF-I concentrations in Angus beef cattle over a 10-year period has shown that elevated serum IGF-I concentrations are only weakly associated with backfat thickness or muscling in postweaning bulls and heifers.

Multiple locus markers are genetic markers that occur in multiple sites throughout the genome. An ideal multiple locus marker is one that is spread throughout the genome, occurring at regular, equal distances on all chromosomes. The multiple locus markers used for molecular markers are highly polymorphic, existing as several different sizes of repetitive DNA fragments, for example, $[-GT-]_n$, $[-GACA-]_n$ or $[-CTCTGGGTGTGGTGC-]_n$. The presence of these variable tandem repeats is revealed by treatment of isolated DNA with restriction endonucleases or by amplification of specific sequences using PCR. In contrast to single locus markers, multiple locus markers do not code for proteins. These repetitive sequences are found in regions of DNA called satellite DNA, either as mini-satellite DNA, consisting of repeats of two to ten bases, or micro-satellite DNA, which consists of 16 to 33 base repeats sequences. The multiple locus markers are used in linkage analyses to examine the inheritance of quantitative trait loci (QTL). QTL are composed of many genes that work in concert to regulate complex production traits such as growth rate, milk and wool production or body composition. Association of QTL with specific multiple locus markers provides a method to indirectly examine the heritability of these complex multigene characteristics. Multilocus marker patterns are specific to individuals and are used as DNA fingerprints to identify individuals, pedigrees, paternity and genetic diseases.

Nutrition

A great deal of time, effort and money has been spent studying the nutritional requirements of animals and the effects of nutrients on animal growth, composition and production. Animal nutrition is a major focus of the animal science curriculum and only cursory comments are given here. Providing the optimal amounts of nutrient to fulfil an animal's requirements results in a healthy animal with good production characteristics. In the context of a specific genetic background, adequate nutrition is required to obtain optimal growth and reach the animal's genetic potential. Adequate amounts of protein, carbohydrate, fat, vitamins and minerals are needed to attain the full genetic potential of an animal. In addition, specific growth promoters such as iodine, calcium, zinc, cobalt and vitamins, as well as the essential amino acids lysine and tryptophan and the essential fatty acids linoleic, linolenic and arachidonic acid are required for optimal growth of animals. The amount and quality of feed is the most important factor in regulating growth rate. Growth is halted or retarded by limiting feed intake. This is, in general, a reversible process and growth will resume if adequate food is returned to the animal. However, if severe nutritional inadequacies are present during early development, permanent stunting of animal size will result. Total available energy intake is the most important dietary component in growth variation. Energy intake can be altered by poor animal health, environmental factors and micronutrient availability. Specific nutrient deficiencies, for example zinc or sodium deficiency, will reduce the feed intake of animals.

Environmental factors

The primary environmental factors that affect animal growth and development are temperature extremes, either heat or cold, and photoperiod effects. While other factors such as arid or humid climates and high altitudes also affect animal health and production, they will not be considered in this section. Photoperiod can be defined as the biphasic change in light intensity or the hours of light vs dark to which an animal is exposed on a daily basis. Photoperiod varies with latitude and with yearly seasons and is considered the most reliable and effective indicator of seasonal changes. In wild animals, the photoperiod serves to synchronize nutrient availability with foraging activity and nutrient use. In addition, seasonal changes in day length induce seasonal breeding to ensure that parturition occurs at an appropriate time of year, usually in the springtime. Most photoperiod effects on breeding and growth have been minimized in domestic animals such as cattle and pigs owing to their intensive breeding and selection for optimal growth and, in the case of swine, the use of artificial housing and lighting. Small ruminants, such as sheep and goats, are still strongly seasonal animals whose growth and reproduction are regulated by photoperiod.

In general, increasing the length of time an animal is exposed to light, up to a point, enhances feed intake and growth rates. Increasing light exposure from the normal 8 to 10 h/day to 14 to 16 h increases growth rates by up to 10% in cattle, sheep and poultry when they are maintained under controlled environmental conditions. Continuous exposure to light (23–24 h) has detrimental effects on growth and production. Longer day lengths have no effects on feed consumption or growth rates in pigs. In sheep and cattle, the primary benefit of longer periods of light exposure is to reduce carcass fat while increasing carcass protein.

The differences in an animal's thermal environment have significant effects on growth and production. The wide disparities in climatic environments between the temperate zones and those of the desert, the northern latitudes and equatorial regions provide a wide variety of climates. Many of the problems encountered with farm animals involve the introduction of European breeds of dairy and beef cattle into extremely hot or cold environments. When domestic animals are exposed to extremes of heat or cold, they must expend a greater amount of energy to maintain their body temperatures. This diverts energy away from growth and from the production of meat, milk and progeny. Animals perform best when maintained within a thermoneutral temperature range. This is the temperature at which there is only a minimal amount of body heat loss or gain. While the thermoneutral range varies by species a general comfort zone ranges from 20°C to 25°C. When temperatures are below this range, animals must conserve and generate heat, while at temperatures above the thermoneutral range, animals must cool themselves by physiological and behavioural adaptations.

The effects of cold temperatures, or cold stress, are especially pronounced in neonatal animals. Exposure of the newborn to low temperatures during the first 72 h of life greatly increases the morbidity and mortality of these animals. Cold stress and the accompanying reduced nutrient intake can increase neonatal mortality rates by 25% to 50% and is obviously an important factor in reproductive success. Animals that are smaller at birth are more susceptible to cold stress due to their reduced capacity for thermogenesis (heat production). Smaller animals also have a relatively larger surface area in relation to their body weight, providing a greater exposed area for heat loss. Thus, twin and triplet lambkins and runt piglets are especially susceptible to cold stress.

The effects of cold stress on growth and production characteristics are especially prominent in swine. Perhaps the most obvious behavioural response to cold stress is an increase in food consumption. This provides the energy for metabolism and thermogenesis so that an animal can maintain a constant body temperature in a cold environment that fosters heat loss. A reduction of external temperature of only 1°C is associated with an increase of 1% to 1.5% of feed intake in pigs in the temperature range of 10°C to 25°C. Although the growth rates of domestic pigs are unaffected by temperatures between 8°C and 20°C, increased feed intake reduces the efficiency of feed utilization. While cold stress is, perhaps, less evident in large ruminants, it has a significant effect on feed consumption. For example, feedlot cattle consume 20–30% more feed during winter months in northern latitudes than in summer months. This is accompanied by similar reductions in feed efficiencies (–27% to 37%) and growth rates (–22% to 33%).

Cold stress induces a number of behavioural and physiological changes that result in body heat conservation and heat production. In addition to increased food consumption, peripheral vasoconstriction redirects blood from the periphery to the body core. This retains heat and reduces heat loss due to passive evaporation and heat exchange with the environment. Animals exposed to cold temperatures huddle together to share body heat and reduce exposed surface areas. Hair coat thickens and hairs stand erect, while birds fluff their feathers as additional barriers to heat loss. Shivering generates additional heat. Long-term exposure to cold results in anatomical changes. Pigs reared at 12°C develop a more squat, rounded morphology with shorter bodies, limbs, snouts, tails and ears. Fat depots undergo redistribution as the percentage of backfat is increased and internal (leaf) fat is reduced. These morphological and anatomical alterations reduce heat loss by providing insulation and by reducing surface area. The generation of heat production in cold-stressed animals is enhanced by mobilization and metabolism of energy substrates. In addition to enhanced food intake, endogenous energy substrates, in the form of glycogen and fat, are utilized to provide energy for metabolism and heat production.

Elevated environmental temperatures present problems to the animal that mirror those of cold stress. Heat stress problems are especially prominent in European breeds of cattle that have been imported to the hot climates of the tropical, subtropical or equatorial regions of the world. In contrast to cold-stressed animals, in which food consumption is increased, the most important response to heat stress is a reduction in food consumption. This reduction in energy substrate availability results in a reduction of metabolism and utilization of dietary protein. This leads to a protein catabolic rate that exceeds protein synthesis and results in a negative nitrogen balance in the body.

Heat stress generally impairs animal growth characteristics. Growth rates, live weights and dry body weights are all reduced in response to heat stress, while body water content is elevated. As a result of reduced food intake, there is a reduction in anabolic metabolism and an elevated catabolism of fat depots and/or lean body mass. The upper critical temperatures for European cattle are 24–30°C for growth and 21–27°C for milk production. At 30°C, milk production is reduced by about 15%, while at 38°C it is reduced by 30%.

Physiological responses to heat stress are characterized by increased heart rates and peripheral vasodilatation that shunts blood from internal organs to peripheral surfaces where heat is dissipated. This is accompanied by hair and feather flattening for more efficient heat exchange. Evaporative processes that enhance cooling, such as increased shallow respiration rates (panting) to enhance evaporation of water from the lungs, passive evaporation from body surfaces and active water loss by perspiration, also play important roles in dissipating heat. Behavioural alterations include a reduction in physical activity, enhanced water consumption and seeking coolness in shade, water or mud.

References and Further Reading

Batt, R.A.L. (1980) *Influences on Animal Growth and Development*. University Park Press, Baltimore, Maryland, 60 pp.

Berg, R.T. and Butterfield, R.M. (1976) *New Concepts of Cattle Growth*. Halsted Press, New York, 238 pp.

Buttery, P.J., Haynes, N.B. and Lindsay, D.B. (1986) *Control and Manipulation of Animal Growth*. Butterworths, London, 347 pp.

Clutter, A.C., Jiang, R., McCann, J.P. and Buchanan, D.S. (1998) Plasma cholecystokinin-8 in pigs with divergent genetic potential for feed intake and growth. *Domestic Animal Endocrinology* 15, 9–21.

Davis, G.P. and Denise, S.K. (1998) The impact of genetic markers on selection. *Journal of Animal Science* 76, 2331–2339.

Hammond, J. (1955) *Progress in the Physiology of Farm Animals*, Vol. 2. Butterworths, London, 740 pp.

Jefferies, A.J., Wilson, V. and Thein, S.L. (1985) Hypervariable minisatellite regions in human DNA. *Nature* 314, 67–73.

Lawrence, T.L.J. and Fowler, V. (2002) *Growth of Farm Animals*, 2nd edn. CAB International, Wallingford, UK, 368 pp.

Phillips, C. and Piggins, D. (1992) *Farm Animals and the Environment*. CAB International, Wallingford, UK, 430 pp.

Scanes, C.G. (2003) *Biology of Growth of Domestic Animals*. Iowa State Press, Ames, Iowa, 408 pp.

Stratz, C.H. (1909) Wachstrum und proportionen des menschen vor und nach der geburt. *Archives in Anthropology* 8, 287–297.

2   Cellular and Molecular Biology

Current biology, whether it is the study of fruit fly genetics or animal science, is often focused at the cellular and molecular levels. It is at this level that further advances in the improvement in production of animals are likely to occur. Thus, a strong background in these concepts is essential to foster the discovery of methods and processes that will alter animal growth, metabolism and production. This chapter presents an outline of the important concepts in molecular and cell biology that are required for an understanding of the processes of animal growth control at the cellular level. While this information may be redundant for some students, it is my experience that many students will benefit from this review. This chapter provides rudimentary information about molecular and cellular mechanisms, with an emphasis on eukaryotic cells.

Prokaryotic and Eukaryotic Organisms

Two broad categories of organisms encompass the range of life. Prokaryotic organisms, the bacteria and archaeobacteria, are comparatively simple, single-celled organisms. They differ fundamentally from the eukaryotic organisms of fungi, plants and animals. Most eukaryotes are multicellular organisms, although a few are single-celled. Multicellular eukaryotes are composed of many different cell types which are specialized for different functions and the cells of eukaryotic organisms are much larger than those of prokaryotes. The structure and functions of eukaryotic cells are much more complex than those of prokaryotic cells. The most distinguishing characteristic of eukaryotic cells is the presence of a nucleus (Greek: *karyon* means kernel or nucleus) and other membranous organelles. Prokaryotic cells have no distinct nucleus, while eukaryotic cells contain a nucleus that is separated from the cytoplasm of the cell by a nuclear membrane. In addition, eukaryotic cells have distinct chromosomes composed of DNA that forms a complex with proteins called histones. This combination of DNA and protein is called chromatin. Prokaryotes, on the other hand, have a single, naked strand of circular DNA without the associated protein coating. The DNA in the nucleus of eukaryotes consists of 10^7 to over 10^{10} base pairs (bp), arranged in a linear fashion, interrupted by non-coding regions called introns. Prokaryotic DNA is much smaller, containing less than 5×10^6 bp, has no introns and is found in the cytoplasm. Finally, eukaryotic cells have a cytoskeleton, composed of polymers of actin that form filaments and microtubules. These provide mechanical support for the cell and allow intracellular movement of organelles. Prokaryotes depend on a rigid cell wall, similar to that of the plants, to support the cell and maintain its shape.

Eukaryotic cell organelles

In the eukaryotic cell, multiple intracellular structures made of membranes are organized to form organelles that are absent in prokaryotic cells. The presence of intracellular organelles in eukaryotes results in a compartmentalization of the cell and a consequent physical isolation of various cell processes (Fig. 2.1). The *plasma membrane* surrounding the eukaryotic cell consists of a hydrophobic lipid bilayer that forms a permeability barrier around the cell. This prevents the free flow of ions and water-soluble molecules between the cell and its external environment. Consequently, molecules entering and leaving the cell do so under regulated processes. The uptake and release of ions such as sodium and potassium are regulated by energy-dependent transport processes, using ATP as an energy source. These processes maintain cellular ionic balance and the electrical potential across the cell membrane of the cell. Likewise, glucose enters the cell by a transmembrane transport molecule. Of importance for hormones, the plasma membrane also contains cell-specific transmembrane hormone

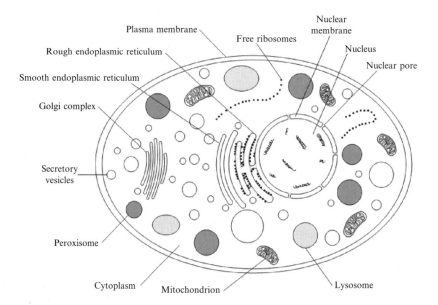

Fig. 2.1. Eukaryotic cell organelles.

receptors that act to bind circulating hormones, transduce their presence through the cell membrane and activate cytoplasmic second messengers. These messengers act as couriers of the hormone signal from the extracellular environment to the nucleus of the cell, resulting in an alteration of gene expression and cellular metabolism.

Eukaryotic organelles are intracellular membranous structures with distinct functions that exist in multiple forms. The *nucleus* is segregated from the cytoplasm by the nuclear membrane, which surrounds and separates the genetic material (genes and chromosomes) from the cytoplasm. It consists of a double membrane interspersed with nuclear pores that allow diffusion of chemicals and communication between the nucleus and the cytoplasm. In the cytoplasm, the *endoplasmic reticulum* is a closed system of sac-like cavities and tubes made of a surrounding membrane. *Rough endoplasmic reticulum* (RER) has many *ribosomes* attached to it, giving it a roughened appearance in cells. This is where proteins are synthesized for insertion into membranes, lysosomes or export from the cell. *Smooth endoplasmic reticulum* (SER) has no associated ribosomes and synthesizes proteins for use within cells, either as soluble nuclear or cytoplasmic proteins or membrane-associated proteins. The SER is also the site of drug metabolism in liver cells and steroid synthesis in endocrine cells. The presence of a signal peptide determines whether a protein is synthesized in the cytoplasm by free ribosomes or in the RER. The *signal peptide* is an amino-terminal 16 to 60 amino acid extension of a protein. This is the first part of the protein that is synthesized. All protein synthesis is initiated in the cytoplasm on free ribosomes. If the signal peptide is present in the newly formed ribosomal-bound peptide, the peptide binds to a signal recognition particle. The particle, the ribosome and its attached immature protein are translocated to the RER. The ribosome attaches to specific receptors on the RER and the signal peptide passes through the membrane of the RER, and leads the growing polypeptide into the lumen of the RER. The signal peptide is cleaved within the RER and the protein enters lysosomal or secretory vesicles.

Like the endoplasmic reticulum, the *Golgi apparatus* is a network of membrane-bound cavities and spaces, arranged in stacks within the cytoplasm. This is the site of protein maturation and protein sorting. The Golgi apparatus receives newly synthesized proteins from the RER and, in a process called post-translational modification, adds sugars to the protein chain to form glycoproteins. The modified proteins are then transported in vesicles to lysosomes, the plasma membrane or to secretory vesicles for release from the cell. *Lysosomes* are vesicles that contain catabolic enzymes for hydrolysis of macromolecules. *Peroxisomes* are membrane-bound organelles that contain enzymes, which use oxygen as an oxidizing agent and produce hydrogen peroxide as a by-product. They are responsible for detoxification of chemicals such as ethanol, phenols and formaldehyde. Peroxisomes are also important in the degradation of long-chain fatty acids via the β-oxidation pathway. Like mitochondria, peroxisomes reproduce by division. *Mitochondria* are small, double-membraned organelles found in almost all eukaryotic cells in large numbers. Mitochondria contain their own DNA,

which is circular and not associated with histones. This DNA is used to synthesize a small proportion of mitochondrial proteins, although most mitochondrial proteins are derived from nuclear genes. Mitochondria provide
the metabolic energy, in the form of ATP, to cells and are most abundant in
cells with extensive oxidative metabolism. Mitochondria are the site of the
oxidative degradation of food within the cell. Oxidative phosphorylation,
the conversion of pyruvate to acetyl-coenzyme A (acetyl-CoA), the citric acid
cycle and the respiratory chain that produces ATP, all occur in the mitochondria. Fatty acid degradation, via the process of β-oxidation, occurs in
the mitochondria. Mitochondria are capable of self-replication and are inherited by offspring only from the maternal parent.

The Cell Cycle

As a eukaryotic cell undergoes mitosis, it must accomplish two things. It
must first double the amount of DNA in its nucleus and then it must halve
this amount of DNA. These processes occur as the cell passes through
defined functional states, called the cell cycle (Fig. 2.2). In all, cell division
in mammals takes anywhere from 10 to 24 h depending on the cell. A 24-h
cell cycle will be used in the example given here. The two basic portions of
a cell's life are mitosis (M) and interphase. Mitosis entails the formation of
microscopically visible chromosomes and their separation into daughter
cells. Due to the visible nature of the chromosomes, mitosis was once the
focus of many cell studies and has been well documented. While important,
mitotic events are only a small part of the cell's life cycle. What was once
called the 'resting' phase, or interphase, when the chromosomes are not visible, is now known to be the time at which cell metabolism and specialized
functions occur. The events that occur during interphase are now called the
cell cycle. The cell cycle consists of distinct portions in which DNA synthe-

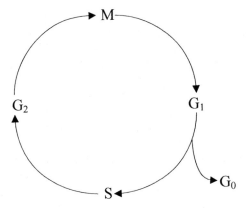

Fig. 2.2. The cell cycle.

sis and the doubling of DNA content occurs, organelles are replicated and attainment and expression of the differentiated state of the cell are apparent.

M: In this phase the formation and separation of visible chromosomes and production of daughter cells occurs. Mitosis is divided into the sequential phases, prophase, metaphase, anaphase and telophase, in which the chromosomes condense, pair and separate. This is followed by cytokinesis, the separation of the cytoplasm and the formation of two daughter cells. In cells grown *in vitro*, mitosis lasts about an hour.

G_1: Originally called a 'gap' phase between mitosis and the S phase, this is the first cell growth phase after mitosis. In this portion of the cell cycle, the cell grows and carries out normal metabolism. This is usually the longest and the most variable part of the cell cycle. It is during this phase that organelles are duplicated. If cells are deficient in nutrients or mitotic signals are absent, this portion of the cell cycle will be prolonged or the cell may enter the G_0 phase and undergo differentiation. In growing cultured cells, this phase lasts 10 h.

G_0: This is the phase in which the cell is 'withdrawn' from the cycle, characterized by active protein synthesis and, in some, motility. This is the phase in which differentiated cells exist. It may last indefinitely or, under appropriate conditions, such as stimulation by mitotic growth factors, the cells may re-enter the cell cycle in the G_1 phase to undergo mitosis.

S: The synthetic phase, when DNA synthesis and chromosome duplication occurs. This phase lasts 8 h.

G_2: This is the second gap, or growth, phase in which the cell grows and prepares for mitosis. Newly replicated DNA is checked for damage and errors in duplication and repaired if necessary. This phase lasts 12 h.

The cell cycle is under the control of regulatory proteins that are activated and inactivated at specific times during the cycle. These regulatory proteins are enzymes called kinases, which phosphorylate specific proteins, and phosphatases, which remove phosphate groups from proteins. The kinases are combinations of two different subunits that are activated by associating with one another to form heterodimers. The regulatory subunit of this heterodimer is called cyclin and the catalytic subunit is called a cyclin-dependent kinase, or Cdk. Concentrations of Cdks are relatively constant throughout the cycle, but cyclin concentrations fluctuate with the phase of the cycle. Thus, the abundance of specific regulatory subunits of the kinases determines the activity of these enzymes. After a specific phase of the cell cycle is completed, the cyclins are dephosphorylated and degraded by the ubiquitin proteolytic system of the cell. There are specific cyclins and Cdks for each stage of the cell cycle. Cyclin D and Cdk4 are present in the G_1 phase and initiate the preparation of chromosomes for replication. Cyclin A and Cdk2 prepare the cell for DNA synthesis of the S phase. In the G_2 phase, the mitotic cyclins, cyclins A and B, associate with Cdk1 to initiate events associated with the beginning of mitosis, such as chromosome condensation and nuclear membrane breakdown.

The Central Dogma of Cell Biology

The central dogma of cell biology is the fundamental basis of cell and molecular biology. This can be summarized by three tenets: (i) DNA can self-replicate (semiconservative replication); (ii) DNA acts as the template for RNA formation (a process called RNA transcription); and (iii) mRNA acts as the template for the synthesis of protein (a process called protein translation). These processes are outlined in Fig. 2.3.

The central dogma of cell biology forms the basis of all processes that occur within the cell, and hence, within the living organism. It includes the replication of DNA so that new cells can be formed, the synthesis of mRNA from specific genes and the translation of the genetic message in RNA into proteins that serve as functional macromolecules within the cell and as messengers between cells. In addition, factors external to the cell, such as hormones and nutrition, as well as innate, endogenous genetic messages, can modulate any of these processes. Regulation of these fundamental processes stimulates mitosis, cell enlargement and accumulation of protein. Altering gene expression of mRNA and subsequently, protein, results in changes in the amount of enzymes and other active proteins present in cells. It is also the basis for the synthesis of proteins for export from the cells, such as secreted factors that regulate the function of other cells, hormones and growth factors. Accumulated proteins and secreted proteins alter the metabolism and thus, function of cells at a particular instant in time or over long periods of time.

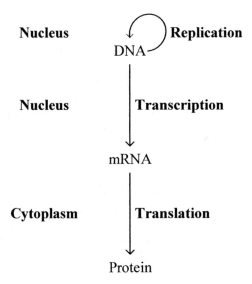

Fig. 2.3. The central dogma of cell biology.

Eukaryotic genes

The function of a structural gene encoding for a specific mRNA is simply to produce a protein. Proteins are diverse molecules, which play many important roles in the cell. As enzymes, proteins catalyse all chemical reactions in the organism. Proteins may act as receptors that mediate hormone actions. Proteins can also be hormones, which modulate the body's response to nutritional, environmental and genetic factors. Structural proteins such as collagen, actin and myosin provide the shape and locomotion for cells and organisms. Proteins are thus essential for the maintenance and regulation of functions in the living organism. The unique sequence of amino acids that defines a protein is coded by the heritable genes in chromosomes of the nucleus. In turn, the overall three-dimensional structure of proteins, which determines their biological role in the animal, results from the unique amino acid sequence of the protein chain. Thus, the properties of these important regulatory and functional molecules are embedded in the genes of an organism.

The genes of eukaryotes are contained within the chromosomes of these organisms. The chromosomes are densely packed structures consisting of DNA and associated proteins, including histones and other proteins. These proteins provide regulatory functions and serve to physically condense the genetic information into a compact form that can be contained within the nucleus. There are about 3 billion pairs of nucleotides (bp) in the human genome, arranged into 46 chromosomes. Each chromosome contains a single molecule of DNA that stretches from one end of the chromosome to the other. Only 5% of this DNA codes for the protein products of expressed genes. This is in contrast to prokaryotes, in which 90% of the DNA codes for proteins. Much of the non-coding DNA in eukaryotes consists of repeated sequences of nucleotides, called interspersed DNA and satellite DNA. The function of non-coding DNA is largely unknown. It may do nothing specifically, simply representing the accumulation of innocuous nonsense DNA over millions of years that is tolerated as long as it does not interrupt the function of essential protein-coding genes. Some non-coding repetitive DNA may play an as yet, unknown regulatory function, altering the expression or silencing of protein-coding genes. Table 2.1 shows the sizes of the genome in various species. The size of an organism's genome varies widely and has no relationship to the perceived complexity of the organism. The mammalian cell contains 5 to 10 pg of DNA, consisting of 3 to 5 billion bp of nucleotides and roughly 30,000 to 50,000 genes.

Genes are transcribed (rewritten) into RNA by enzymes called RNA polymerases, which move from the 5′ to the 3′ end of the DNA. While a prokaryotic gene that codes for a specific mRNA consists of continuous coding sequence of DNA, eukaryotic genes coding for mRNA are discontinuous, with large sections of interspersed non-coding DNA (Fig. 2.4). Eukaryotic genes are composed of stretches of DNA called exons (expressed regions) that encode for mRNA. Non-coding sections of DNA, called introns (intervening regions), separate exons from one another. Introns can range in

Table 2.1. Sizes of the genome in base pairs (bp) and number of chromosomes of various species.

Species	bp	Chromosomes
Human	3.5×10^9	23
Bovine	3×10^9	60
Mouse	3×10^9	40
Chicken	2.1×10^9	78
Frog	4.5×10^{10}	26
Maize	5×10^{10}	10
Drosophila	1.6×10^8	8
Saccharomyces cerevisiae (yeast)	1.4×10^7	34
Escherichia coli	4×10^6	1

size from 75 to 10,000 nucleotides. The average mammalian gene contains eight introns, but can contain more than 50 of these non-coding regions within a gene. Some of the non-coding intron regions play a part in the regulation of gene expression. A promoter region, located upstream (5′) to the gene to be transcribed, consists of specific sequences of DNA to which RNA polymerase II and other protein factors needed for gene transcription bind. This is the area where gene transcription is initiated. The 5′ and 3′ flanking regions of the gene contain distant regulatory elements that bind protein transcription factors that enhance or suppress gene expression.

When genes are transcribed into mRNA, both introns and exons are copied. The introns are then removed with specific enzymes by a process called pre-mRNA splicing. This results in a mature mRNA that contains only exons that is translated into protein (see later). The interrupted genes of eukaryotes provide a way in which multiple mRNA and protein products can be produced from a single gene, increasing the number and diversity of

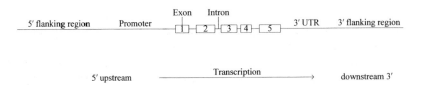

Fig. 2.4. Eukaryotic gene structure. The 5′ and 3′ flanking regions and the 3′ untranslated region contain enhancer regions and response elements that regulate gene activity.

proteins produced by a gene. Many genes contain more than one promoter site where gene transcription can begin. This results in some protein products that may be slightly larger (or smaller) than others. In addition, after transcription, different combinations of exons may result due to alternate splicing of the mRNA. That is, differential splicing of exons to one another can result in the formation of multiple mRNAs from a single gene. Thus, a gene may produce an mRNA that consists of, for example, exons 1, 2 and 3 or exons 1, 2 and 4. The resulting proteins are closely related isoforms of one another, but one form may have enhanced biological activity or may appear only in a specific tissue.

Ribonucleic Acid

RNA has many functions in the cell. Messenger RNA contains the code for the amino acid sequence of the mature protein, transfer RNA carries specific amino acids that are used in protein synthesis and ribosomal RNA provides the catalytic centre of protein synthesis on ribosomes. The sizes of the RNAs are often given as sedimentation coefficients (S), which relate to the rate of movement, or sedimentation, of a molecule in a centrifugal field. Three general types of RNA are present in cells:

1. Ribosomal RNA (rRNA) is a structural and catalytic RNA, which together with about 85 different proteins, forms the ribosomes. It is the most abundant RNA in the cell, comprising about 75% of total cellular RNA. In eukaryotes, rRNA exists in four forms: 18S RNA, 28S RNA, 5.8S RNA and 5S RNA.
2. Transfer RNA (tRNA) and small nuclear RNAs are small, stable RNAs. tRNA consists of about 75 nucleotides and is responsible for amino acid transfer during protein synthesis. Small nuclear RNA (snRNA) has enzymatic activity and is involved in RNA splicing.
3. Messenger RNA (mRNA) is the copy of a gene that codes for a specific protein. It is initially transcribed as a large precursor molecule, called heterogeneous nuclear RNA (hnRNA). HnRNA is enzymatically cleaved by snRNA to remove introns and to form mature mRNA. Messenger RNA is only a small portion of cellular RNA comprising less than 5% of total RNA in the cell.

Messenger RNA and translation of protein

Transcription of protein-coding genes results in large hnRNA, containing introns and exons of the gene. The introns are enzymatically removed from the hnRNA and the remaining exons spliced together to mature mRNA molecule. Messenger RNA of eukaryotic cells undergoes further modifications that result in several unique characteristics (Fig. 2.5). The 5' end of the molecule, where translation is initiated, is capped by methylation of the guanosine molecule. This provides protection from phosphatase and 5'

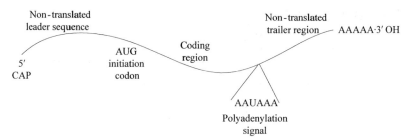

Fig. 2.5. Anatomy of the messenger RNA molecule.

exonuclease degradation. A leader sequence, also called the 5′ untranslated region (UTR), follows the 5′ end of the molecule. This 30- to 50-nucleotide stretch is thought to provide proper alignment with the protein synthetic material. The coding region, consisting of triplet nucleotides, which each code for a single amino acid, usually has an initial AUG (Met) codon as the translation initiation sequence.

At the end of the coding region, nonsense codons (UAA, UAG or UGA) signal the termination of translation. The trailer sequence (also called the 3′ UTR) follows. This consists of 50 to 150 nucleotides and may provide stability to the mRNA. Within this region is the AAUAAA sequence, which codes for addition of the polyA tail. The 3′ end of the mRNA molecule has a characteristic polyadenylic acid (polyA) sequence of 50 to 250 adenosines. This occurs in 97% of all mRNA species, although the mRNA which codes for chromatin protein histone (~30% of all mRNA) is not polyadenylated. The polyA tail is believed to protect against 3′ exonucleases and may enhance translational efficiency.

Translation of mRNA into the final protein product occurs in the cell's cytoplasm and involves the interaction of mRNA, tRNA and ribosomes. The information coded in mRNA consists of groups of three bases, called codons, each specifying a particular amino acid (Table 2.2). These codons are recognized by complementary triplet bases, the anticodon, located on the tRNA molecule. Transfer RNAs carry specific amino acids specified by the anticodon–codon to the mRNA. Ribosomes are large macromolecular structures that coordinate the interaction between mRNA and tRNA to synthesize a protein or polypeptide. These large structures consist of rRNA core and over 85 small, basic, surface proteins surrounding the rRNA. A eukaryotic ribosome has an overall size of 80S and consists of two subunits, a large 60S subunit that contains 28S, 5S and 5.8S rRNA and a smaller 40S subunit that contains 18S rRNA. Translating the mRNA sequence into a protein chain takes place in the space between the two ribosomal subunits. The process of protein translation involves the initiation of the process by binding to the initiation codon (AUG) of the mRNA, followed by chain elongation in the order specified by the mRNA codon, and finally chain termination at termination codons (UAA, UAG or UGA), when translation stops, and the ribosomal subunits dissociate.

Table 2.2. The genetic code.

First base (5'end)	Second base				Third base (3'end)
	U	C	A	G	
U	Phe	Ser	Tyr	Cys	U
	Phe	Ser	Tyr	Cys	C
	Leu	Ser	Ter	Ter	A
	Leu	Ser	Ter	Trp	G
C	Leu	Pro	His	Arg	U
	Leu	Pro	His	Arg	C
	Leu	Pro	Gln	Arg	A
	Leu	Pro	Gln	Arg	G
A	Ile	Thr	Asn	Ser	U
	Ile	Thr	Asn	Ser	C
	Ile	Thr	Lys	Arg	A
	Met	Thr	Lys	Arg	G
G	Val	Ala	Asp	Gly	U
	Val	Ala	Asp	Gly	C
	Val	Ala	Glu	Gly	A
	Val	Ala	Glu	Gly	G

RNA polymerases

Three types of RNA polymerase enzymes catalyse the transcription of RNA from DNA. RNA polymerase I transcribes tandem repeat ribosomal RNA genes located in the nucleolus to produce 18S, 28S and 5.8S RNAs, structural components of rRNA. RNA polymerase II transcribes all protein-coding genes to form mRNA. In addition, RNA polymerase II catalyses the formation of most snRNAs involved in RNA splicing. The formation of tRNA and 5S RNA is catalysed by RNA polymerase III.

Transcription of genes by RNA polymerases I and III is relatively straightforward. These polymerases catalyse the formation of large quantities of rRNA and tRNA, respectively. These are relatively homogeneous species of RNA that are not translated into proteins. There is only a single promoter for the transcription of rRNA genes by RNA polymerase I and transcription of tRNA genes is regulated by two promoters.

RNA polymerase II, on the other hand, is responsible for catalysing the transcription of thousands of different genes, each coding for different proteins in the cell. A single cell may contain 10,000 to 20,000 different mRNAs, each present in widely different concentrations, which vary by tissue and during different developmental and metabolic stages. Thus, the differential and specific transcription of multiple, unique, genes by RNA polymerase II is complex. This process is highly regulated by interactions of RNA polymerase with specific nuclear proteins that assist in assuring that genes are expressed appropriately.

Regulation of gene transcription

Compared to prokaryotes, eukaryotic genes are relatively complex. Eukaryotic genes consist of the gene itself and several regulatory gene elements that flank the protein-coding part of the gene. All cells of a plant or animal contain exactly the same genes, but cells use only a small subset of these genes. The control of gene transcription is initiated in the promoter region of the gene, located upstream (5′) to the gene itself. The promoter is defined as the DNA sequences needed to initiate gene transcription. The promoter region binds RNA polymerase and other regulatory proteins necessary to initiate transcription. The regulation of gene expression is under control of regulatory proteins that bind to regulatory elements in the promoter and activate or inhibit gene transcription. These proteins are called transcription factors and they bind to other proteins and to specific sequences in the promoter region of the gene called control elements. When a transcription factor inhibits transcription, it is called a repressor and if a transcription factor stimulates transcription it is called an inducer or activator.

Genes can be classified as those that are always active, producing gene products at a basal state, and those in which transcription is regulated. Genes that are constantly transcribed are those that code for structural proteins of the cell and those involved with cell metabolism. These basal, constitutively active genes are called housekeeping genes. On the other hand, regulated genes are activated or repressed only during specific metabolic processes. These would include genes regulated during cell growth and differentiation, or in response to specific stimuli, such as hormone activation or cell stress. The focus here is on regulated genes that respond to changes in the cell environment.

The promoter region of most genes that code for proteins contains a DNA sequence called the *TATA box*, with the sequence TATAA. This sequence is located at the 3′ end of the promoter region, about 30 bases upstream from the transcription initiation site of many genes. This is the element that binds RNA polymerase II. However, polymerase II by itself cannot initiate transcription. A basal level of transcription requires the presence of several transcription factors along with RNA polymerase II. These are called *general transcription factors* (GTF) and over 20 of them have been discovered. The initiation of gene transcription requires the ordered, sequential assembly of six of these GTFs into a macromolecular aggregate with RNA polymerase II. The first of these GTFs is called the TATA box-binding protein (TBP). This factor is common to all three polymerases and can help to initiate transcription in genes regulated by RNA polymerases I, II and III. The initial assembly of the transcription complex for genes transcribed by RNA polymerase II involves the binding of TBP to other proteins to form the transcription factor TFIID, which binds to the TATA box and opens the double-stranded DNA. Binding of other factors TFIIA and TFIIB provides stability to the complex and assures the selection of the correct transcription start site. It is only now that RNA polymerase II, bound to another transcription factor (TFIIF), binds to the TATA box. The final GTFs involved in the initiation of basal transcription, TFIIE and TFIIH, provide the final components of the transcription apparatus (Fig. 2.6). From this brief description, it is apparent that initiation of basal transcription involves the cooperation of a variety of regulatory proteins to provide the efficient transcription of a gene.

Transcriptional control of specific genes

Control of the transcription of specific genes involves additional regulatory elements. While the general transcriptional elements and associated proteins can induce limited expression of a gene, the full activation of gene expression requires other promoter elements. There are two types of elements: proximal promoter elements (PPE) and enhancer elements. The PPE are located near the gene, 50 to 250 bp upstream from the transcriptional start site. These are small stretches of DNA (<10 bp) that bind additional regulatory proteins. Two important examples of PPEs are the CAT box, with the sequence CCAAT, and the SP1 site, with the sequence GGCGCC. Both sites are present in many housekeeping genes and are required for full transcriptional activity. Most promoters have many different PPEs, also called response elements, which respond to a variety of factors, ranging from metals to transcription factors that mediate the effects of hormones. Thus, specific gene transcription is regulated by the presence of several specific

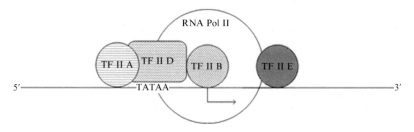

Fig. 2.6. The eukaryotic transcription complex.

response elements associated with a particular gene. The effectiveness of these response elements depends upon the relative availability and activity of multiple protein transcription factors. The presence of PPEs and their associated transcription factors adds another level of regulatory control and complexity to control the expression of genes. This complex array of regulatory elements and their associated transcription factors assures a fine-tuned response to factors that alter gene expression.

The *enhancer elements* are another type of promoter element that controls gene expression. Enhancer elements are characterized by their ability to affect gene transcription when located at great distances, up to 10 kb, from the gene. Enhancer elements may also be present within the genes themselves, within the introns of genes. They participate in the regulation of many, if not all genes. They are able to regulate gene transcription from great distances as the regulatory proteins that bind to them also bind to other proteins attached to distant sites on DNA. These protein–protein interactions are possible because of loops in the DNA strand. This allows the physical contact of proteins bound to distant enhancer elements with those near the transcription start site. As their name implies, enhancer sequences interact with transcription factors and enhance the rate of specific gene transcription, although they cannot initiate transcription by themselves. Enhancer elements for tissue-specific transcription factors confer transcriptional regulation on a tissue-specific basis.

Transcription factors

Hundreds of gene-specific transcription factors have been discovered since the 1990s. It is estimated that approximately 6% of the human genome (total DNA) is devoted to the production of these proteins. Despite this abundance, the regulation of specific gene transcription involves not a single unique transcription factor, but requires different combinations, specific to each gene, of several of these proteins. Although most of these transcription factors are activators of gene transcription, repressors have also been identified.

Transcription factors are classified based upon the structure of their specific DNA-binding domains. There are three basic types:

1. *Homeodomain proteins* contain a conserved 60 amino acid domain (the homeobox) and a helix–turn–helix domain. Both domains interact with specific DNA sequences. There are more than 150 of these transcription factors in humans. Many homeodomain proteins play important roles in the development of embryonic structures such as the muscles, limbs and nervous system.

2. *Zinc finger proteins* contain multiple polypeptide 'fingers' consisting conserved pairs of cysteines and histidines that bind a single zinc ion. More than 600 of these proteins exist in humans. The tip of the zinc finger interacts with bases in DNA. Steroid nuclear receptors, which contain a specific ligand-binding domain for steroid attachment and a DNA-binding domain, are in this category of transcription factors.

3. *Leucine zipper proteins* contain a basic amino acid region that binds to DNA and a series of repeated leucine residues. The leucine repeats form an α-helix that binds other leucine zipper molecules to form a dimer. An important regulatory transcription factor that initiates adipose tissue formation, called CAAT/enhancer-binding protein (C/EBP), is an example of a leucine zipper protein. Basic helix–loop–helix (bHLH) proteins are similar to leucine zipper proteins but have two dimerization domains separated by a loop region. The muscle regulatory factors (MRFs), such as MyoD, that induce muscle differentiation are examples of bHLH transcription factors.

Biotechnology and Genetic Engineering

Biotechnology is defined as the use of technologies based upon living systems to develop commercial processes and products – making a buck from biology. Some examples of biotechnology directed toward animal production systems include gene transfer to produce transgenic animals that contain a foreign gene that may enhance growth or the production of animal products such as meat, milk or fibre. The processes of embryo manipulation and tissue culture are also considered as biotechnological processes. Biotechnology is used for bioprocess engineering, in which production of specific animal proteins using bacterial or mammalian cell cultures is accomplished. The process of producing monoclonal antibodies is a large and important field of biotechnology. Monoclonal antibodies are produced from immortalized clones of antibody-producing lymphocytes. As such, these antibodies are very specific for their antigen targets and are used for the diagnosis and prevention of many diseases.

The relatively recent explosion in the use of biotechnology after the 1980s has come about because of discoveries in the chemistry and manipulation of genes at the molecular level. The production of complex proteins containing hundreds of amino acids in the proper sequence cannot be done economically or efficiently using synthetic organic chemistry methods. Instead, a living system, bacterial or eukaryotic, must be involved in the sequential ordering of amino acids to form a biologically active, functional protein. For this purpose, recombinant DNA is produced. A simple definition of recombinant DNA is that DNA from one source recombined with DNA from another, often bacterial or viral, source.

Introduction of a specific gene that codes for a particular protein has many uses. After introduction of a gene into a bacterium, the bacteria can be grown *en masse* to amplify the foreign gene. That gene can then be used in the production of specific proteins, either *in vivo* or *in vitro*. After removal of the amplified foreign gene from the bacteria, it can be used to produce transgenic plants or animals with the goal of improving agricultural production. About 70% of the soybeans and cotton that are grown in the USA are now derived from transgenic organisms, as is 30% of the US maize crop. Many of the transgenic plants are engineered to be resistant to the glyphosate herbicide Roundup® or to contain the naturally occurring insecticide *Bacillus thuringiensis* toxin gene for resistance to insects. A more ambitious goal for human medicine is to use specific genes to correct diseases of genetic origin.

Transgenic Animals and their Potential

Only since the mid-1970s have we been able to isolate specific genes, sequence them and recombine them with the DNA of foreign hosts. The importance of the ability to make specific proteins cannot be overemphasized. Knowing the genetic code for amino acids and proteins allows them to be modified – 'nature improved upon' amino acid sequences can be changed to reduce degradation (increase half-life) of proteins, increase the efficiency of enzymes, or to increase hormone/receptor efficiency.

In the context of animal agriculture, animals produced with an added gene can be used to improve productivity (produce more meat, fibre or milk with less or the same nutrient intake), as measured by growth rate, feed efficiency, milk efficiency, wool production or reproductive efficiency. An example of the latter is the potential to increase twin lambs in sheep by introducing the Booroola gene for twinning. Insertion of antibody genes to enhance immune function to a specific disease might be used to induce disease resistance of animals. In addition, transgenic animals that express a specific gene into an easily accessible compartment, such as milk, allows the animal to be used as a 'bioreactor', capable of producing a specific protein. This has the advantage of high-yield productions in a mammalian host that would lack possible bacterial toxins that may be present in recombinant products isolated from bacterial cultures. Introduction of specific genes, for example the gene for GH or leptin, has the potential to alter body composition by increasing lean body deposition with a reduction in body fat. Alteration of the ruminant microbial genome has the potential to alter the efficiency of rumenal digestion. Transgenic animals provide the opportunity for 'instant evolution', as the introduced gene or genes are incorporated into all cells of the body, including the germ line cells. Thus, dramatic, heritable changes may be introduced into an animal and, if successful, could save generations of breeding and selection for favourable traits.

Identifying, Isolating and Transferring Genes

The mammalian genome has about 3 to 4 billion bp of DNA. Of this number, there are about 35,000 to 50,000 genes that code for protein products. As a single gene consists of 1000 to 5000 bases, this accounts for less than 10% of the total genomic DNA. Most estimates suggest that ~95% of genomic DNA does not code for proteins. The majority of DNA is believed to be regulatory in nature, assuring that genes are expressed at the proper time in development, by a specific cell and in response to a specific environmental cue. When cellular RNA is considered, only a small proportion of the total RNA is devoted to mRNA that codes for proteins. Roughly 2% to 5% of cellular RNA is mRNA, while the rest is transfer and ribosomal RNA. With this knowledge, it is apparent that the isolation of a single specific gene from this tangle of DNA is a Herculean task.

Genes can be isolated in several different ways. Chemical synthesis (if sequence is known) can produce only relatively small pieces of DNA (a few hundred bases, with luck). Another approach is to digest total DNA, using restriction endonucleases (RE), into 15–20 kb fragments. The digested DNA is inserted into plasmids or bacteriophages and grown in the host to amplify the DNA fragments. This is called a genomic library, which consists of thousands of pieces of DNA, mostly non-coding introns and repetitive DNA. This approach is used primarily for DNA sequencing of entire genomes.

The most common approach to the isolation of the gene that codes for a specific protein is to prepare a complementary (cDNA) library. Complementary DNA is a copy of the mRNA present in a specific tissue or cell at a specific time. After isolation of total RNA from the organ or tissue of interest, the mRNA fraction is isolated by binding to a synthetic polyT resin, either in an aqueous column or in a test tube. As the majority of mRNA has a polyA sequence that is complementary to the polyT sequence, mRNA will be selectively enriched from the total RNA, thereby eliminating 95% to 99% of the total RNA. Messenger RNA is then subjected to reverse transcription to prepare cDNA from total mRNA. The cDNA is then introduced into bacterial plasmids (or bacteriophages) and amplified by growing the recombinant organisms *in vitro*. This is called a cDNA library. It consists of cDNA derived only from the mRNA population of the cell and only the exons of the gene are present. After reintroduction of the recombinant plasmids into the bacteria, the bacteria are allowed to grow, reproducing and amplifying the plasmids. Bacterial colonies containing the genes of interest are then identified and selected with probes that contain sequences complementary to the mRNA of interest. After amplification of the foreign DNA of interest, it is then removed from the plasmid using restriction enzymes, purified and used in an animal (or plant) host to produce a transgenic organism. This process is outlined below.

The use of bacterial RE has allowed the isolation, manipulation and recombination of DNA. RE, also called restriction enzymes, are bacteria's natural defence system that protect the bacterium from viral (bacteriophage) invasion. They protect bacteria by digesting foreign, non-methylated viral DNA, while methylation of bacterial DNA protects it from self-digestion. They are called RE because they restrict the growth of viral bacteriophages in bacterial hosts. Restriction enzymes bind to and cleave DNA at specific sequences. Due to the specific site of 'cutting' and reproducibility of these enzymatic reactions, production of DNA fragments can be controlled and the generation of specific sequences of DNA can be reproducibly performed.

Restriction enzymes are given names that are abbreviations of the bacteria from which they came (Fig. 2.7). Restriction enzymes cut double-stranded

Enzyme abbreviation	Microorganism	Sequence recognized
*Bam*HI	*Bacillus amyloliquefaciens* H	5′...G|GATCC...3′ 3′...CCTAG|G...5′
*Hae*III	*Haemophilus aegytius*	5′...GG|CC...3′ 3′...CC|GG...5′
*Hha*I	*Haemophilus haemolyticus*	5′...GCG|C...3′ 3′...C|GCG...5′
*Dde*I	*Desulfovibrio desulfuricans*	5′...C|T*N*AG...3′ 3′...GA*N*T|C...5′
*Eco*RV	*Escherichia coli*	5′...GAT|ATC...3′ 3′...CTA|TAG...5′
*Eco*RI	*Escherichia coli*	5′...G|AATTC...3′ 3′...CTTAA|G...5′
*Pst*I	*Providencia stuarti*	5′...CTGCA|G...3′ 3′...GA|CGTC...5′
*Mst*II	*Microcoleus*	5′...CC|T*N*AGG...3′ 3′...GGA*N*T|CC...5′

Fig. 2.7. Restriction endonucleases and their sites of action.

DNA at areas with a twofold axis of symmetry. These palindromic sequences have the same sequence from left to right as they do in the reverse order. Examples of language palindromes include, e.g. 'Madam I'm Adam'; 'A man, a plan, a canal, Panama'. Cleavage of double-stranded DNA by restriction enzymes may leave blunt ends, in which the two strands of DNA are cut at the same length, with no extended strands. Other restriction enzymes leave staggered, overlapping ends of DNA on their digested strands. These single-stranded extensions of the DNA molecule are called 'sticky ends' as they are available for complementary (A–T or G–C) hydrogen bonding to form double-stranded DNA (Fig. 2.8). Blunt ends can be enzymatically 'tailed' to introduce restriction enzyme sites and/or sticky ends available for hydrogen bonding.

...GG|CC... —*Hae*III→ ...GG + CC...
...CC|GG... ...CC GG...

Blunt ends

...G|AATTC... —*Eco*RI→ ...G + AATTC...
...CTTAA|G... ...CTTAA G...

Sticky ends

Fig. 2.8. Production of blunt or sticky ends of DNA by restriction endonucleases.

The bacterial chromosome consists of a single circular molecule of 'naked' DNA. In addition, bacteria have small (10^3 to 10^5 bp) circular, auxiliary DNA called plasmids. Plasmids are abundant (20–30+ copies per cell), self-replicating, and are transferred from one bacterium to another. Plasmids are used as the insertion site for the introduction of foreign DNA into bacteria to create recombinant DNA. Bacteriophages, viruses that infect bacteria by injecting their DNA into them, may also be used to introduce foreign DNA into bacteria. Some plasmids carry genes for resistance to antibiotics such as ampicillin or tetracycline. When foreign genes are inserted into the plasmid's antibiotic resistance genes, the resistance genes are disrupted, inducing specific antibiotic susceptibility. This provides a simple method to identify bacteria containing foreign DNA, as the recombinant bacteria, grown in duplicate cultures, are killed by exposure to specific antibiotics. Synthetic plasmids are now widely available commercially which contain inserted RE sites and antibiotic resistance genes. An example of this is the pBR322 plasmid, which contains both ampicillin and tetracycline resistance genes and DNA sequences for specific restriction enzymes (Fig. 2.9). Newer synthetic plasmids are equipped with colour-producing genes for easy identification of foreign gene insertion, so that selection for recombinant clones is simplified.

To make recombinant DNA, both plasmid DNA and isolated foreign cDNA are digested with the same RE, to produce complementary sticky ends. The *Bam*HI enzyme can be used for this as a restriction site for this enzyme disrupts the tetracycline resistance gene of the pBR322 gene (Fig. 2.10). After plasmid and foreign gene DNA are digested with *Bam*HI, they are combined and heated to 70°C to separate the hydrogen-bonded strands. The reaction mixture is then cooled to allow the complementary sticky ends

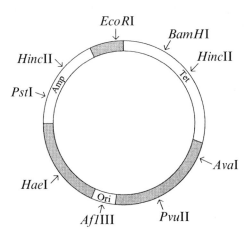

Fig. 2.9. The pBR322 plasmid. Some restriction endonucleases sites (arrows) are shown. Amp, ampicillin resistance gene; Tet, tetracycline resistance gene; Ori, replication origin site.

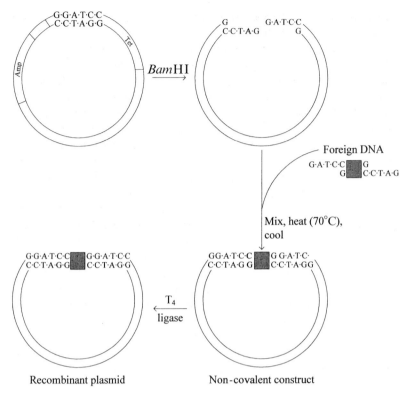

Fig. 2.10. Introduction of foreign DNA into the pBR322 plasmid.

to recombine. When the treatment is complete, unwanted by-products are also formed in addition to the desired plasmid–gene recombinant DNA. These include intact plasmids and intact genes that must be removed from the recombinant DNA. The recombinant DNA at this stage is attached only by non-covalent hydrogen bonds between the complementary bases of the DNA strands of the sticky ends. To covalently incorporate the foreign DNA within the plasmid, the enzyme T_4 ligase is used. The plasmids are reintroduced into bacteria, using either osmotic shock – high calcium (20–50 mM), or electrophoretic transfer (electrophoration) and plated on to an agar growth medium. Bacteria are allowed to grow into visible colonies. The colonies that contain the recombinant DNA are selected using replicate plating – colonies picked up with a felt template and transferred to antibiotic-containing agar – recombinant colonies are identified by their sensitivity to antibiotics, in this case tetracycline, and selected for clonal growth. Alternatively, colony replicates on nitrocellulose paper can be hybridized to complementary, labelled probes specific for the inserted DNA to identify positive colonies. Newer technology uses synthetic plasmids, e.g. pGEM, which contain genes (LacZ = β-galactosidase) that can be detected by colour screening with appropriate substrate. Intact LacZ produces blue colonies.

Positive colonies are then grown in large suspension cultures, plasmids isolated, digested with the restriction enzyme used to produce the original recombinants and the amplified foreign gene is purified.

To introduce the amplified gene into a multicellular animal, it is microinjected into a newly fertilized oocyte, transferred into a foster mother and allowed to come to term. This results in random incorporation of the gene into host chromosomes. There are several problems associated with random incorporation of DNA into the host chromosomes. The success rate is low, ~1% viable transgenics are produced from the injected eggs. The chances of introducing a lethal mutation are high, as the foreign gene may be incorporated into an existing gene that is essential for metabolism. When genes are randomly incorporated into the oocyte, all body cells, somatic and germ line cells, contain and express the gene. When the gene is introduced without appropriate regulatory controls, inappropriate developmental gene expression occurs and the introduced gene is expressed in embryonic, fetal, neonatal and adult animals. The normal developmental, tissue-specific regulation of gene expression is lost and the gene is either fully expressed or not. High levels of unregulated gene products lead to pharmacological effects and metabolic diseases. The hit-or-miss random incorporation of genes leads to low success rates. These problems have been addressed by targeting genes to specific sites in the animal's genome and by adding regulatory elements that restrict gene expression to specific organs during specific developmental stages and in response to specific regulatory signals.

Homologous recombination, gene targeting and gene knockouts

When a foreign gene is introduced into mammalian cells, it is incorporated into DNA at random locations. Most of the time the foreign gene recombines with the host DNA at a site that is unrelated to the introduced gene. This is called heterologous recombination. In a very few instances, about 1 in 1000, the gene recombines with the identical site of the original gene by a process called homologous recombination. Methods to increase rates of homologous recombination of introduced genes or to enrich cell populations that have undergone homologous recombination offer powerful tools to study gene function and to produce transgenic animals that are more physiologically viable. Homologous recombination can be used to target gene insertions to an exact known location in the genome. This provides the potential for gene replacement, in which a functional gene can be used to replace a defective one. In animal production, one can envision the replacement of a naturally occurring gene with one that is genetically engineered, to produce a gene that is more efficiently regulated or one that produces a protein product with enhanced biological activity.

At present, homologous recombination is used primarily to disrupt specific genes in an animal. Animals that have successfully undergone homologous recombination can be produced. Mice are used for this process owing to their abundance, well-known genetics and short generation times.

Animals in which the gene has been disrupted are termed gene knockout mice. This method has provided a powerful tool to study the functions of specific gene products. The gene to be disrupted is modified *in vitro* by the insertion of a selectable marker gene that has no promoter (Fig. 2.11). The marker gene confers drug resistance on the cell and its presence protects the cell from lethal drug effects. A marker commonly used in mammalian cells is a bacterial gene that confers resistance to a neomycin-related drug, G418. This drug kills mammalian cells by inhibiting protein synthesis. The gene is transfected into embryonic stem cells maintained *in vitro*. Embryonic stem cells are undifferentiated pluripotent cells derived from the inner cell mass of the embryonic blastocyst. They are used because of their ability to differentiate into all cell lineages of the animal, including the germ cells that will form spermatozoa and ova. When the promoterless gene is incorporated into its appropriate locus in the genome, the endogenous promoter activates it and the gene product coding for G418 resistance is expressed. Cells without the drug resistance gene die upon exposure to G418 while those that have incorporated the gene via homologous recombination survive. These cells are then isolated, cloned and injected into a blastocyst, which is transplanted into a foster mother and allowed to come to term (Fig. 2.12). Many of the resulting pups are chimeras, containing wild-type cells from the blastocyst and the introduced stem cells. These chimeric animals can be easily identified if one uses embryonic stem cells derived from black mice and donor embryos collected from homozygous white mice, or vice versa. Chimeric animals, containing the modified gene, are characterized by black and white patches of fur. These mice can be screened with probes complementary to the gene of interest to ensure the presence of the appropriate targeted allele and then interbred with animals homozygous for coat colour to produce animals homozygous for the desired mutation.

This method for gene disruption has been refined in recent years to eliminate some of the problems associated with traditional gene-targeting meth-

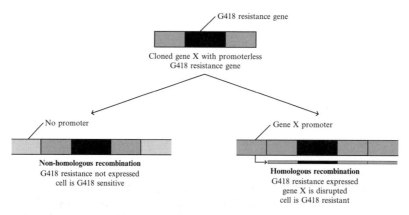

Fig. 2.11. Homologous recombination and gene disruption.

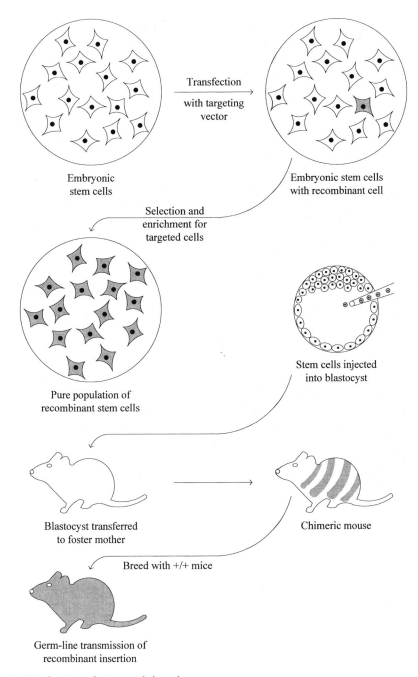

Fig. 2.12. Production of mice with knockout genes.

ods. As with transgenic animals, the disrupted gene is present in all tissues at all stages of development. This can lead to relatively non-specific effects and to embryonic mortality. Tissue-specific or developmentally regulated genes can be disrupted using the Cre-lox recombinase system. Recognition sites on DNA for the Cre-recombinase enzyme, called loxP sites, are inserted into both ends of the gene to be disrupted and transgenic mice with the insertion are produced by injecting the modified gene into embryos. Another set of mice is generated with the Cre-recombinase enzyme linked to tissue-specific promoters. Mating of mice engineered with the flanking loxP sites with those producing the Cre-recombinase enzyme produces animals in which a specific gene is disrupted in a developmental or tissue-specific manner.

Animals produced by these methods have provided valuable tools to study the functional roles of hormones and growth factors. Elimination of specific hormone, growth factor or transcription factor genes produces animals with altered metabolic or developmental traits. Many times, these mutations are lethal and animals die before embryonic and fetal development is complete. In other cases, disruption of specific genes produces a viable animal that is stunted or an animal that is deficient in a specific tissue such as bone, fat or muscle. Knockout mice and their uses will be addressed in subsequent chapters that deal with the development of specific tissues, growth factors and transcription factors.

References and Further Reading

Betz, U.A., Vosshenrich, C.A., Rajewsky, K. and Muller, W. (1996) Bypass of lethality with mosaic mice generated by Cre-loxP-mediated recombination. *Current Biology* 6, 1307–1316.

Capecchi, M.R. (1989) Altering the genome by homologous recombination. *Science* 244, 1288–1292.

Hawkins, J.D. (1985) *Gene Structure and Expression*. Cambridge University Press, Cambridge, UK, 173 pp.

Pollard, T.D. and Earnshaw, W.C. (2002) *Cell Biology*. W.B. Saunders, Elsevier Science, Philadelphia, Pennsylvania, 805 pp.

Novikoff, A.B. and Holtzman, E. (1970) *Cells and Organelles*. Holt, Rinehart and Winston, New York, 337 pp.

Watson, J.D., Gilman, M., Witkowski, J. and Zoller, M. (1992) *Recombinant DNA*, 2nd edn. W.H. Freeman, New York, 626 pp.

3   The Endocrine System

The endocrine system is an essential regulatory component of animal physiology, metabolism and growth. The endocrine system plays a central role in the regulation of nutritional intake and utilization, and integrates the multiple functions of physiological systems. Unlike enzymes, which are secreted into the gastrointestinal tract by glands in the tract, hormones are secreted directly into the bloodstream by a variety of ductless glands located throughout the body.

Starling, in 1905, defined a hormone as a 'chemical messenger which is speeding from cell to cell along the bloodstream, may coordinate the activities and growth of different parts of the body'. Stated differently, we now know that a hormone is a chemical messenger secreted by a discrete, ductless gland directly into the bloodstream, which carries it to its distant, usually well-defined target cells that contain specific hormone receptors, where the hormone elicits a response. Hormones circulate and are active at very low concentrations (10^{-9} to 10^{-12} M). More recently, the definition of a hormone has been broadened, as some hormones that were thought to be confined to a single source are now known to be produced by multiple tissues. For example, the products of the pancreatic islets, the pituitary and thyroid glands were thought to be strictly defined hormones. In the past few years, it has been shown that insulin, glucagon and thyroid hormones are produced at sites distant from their respective glands. These locally produced hormones may stimulate changes in the growth and metabolism of cells without the intervention of the circulatory system. Other examples of hormones, which also act as local growth factors, are the IGFs, leptin and somatostatin (SS). Hormones and growth factors can act in multiple ways, which do not involve the intervention of the circulatory system (Fig. 3.1). Thus, autocrine hormones are those which affect the same cell that produced them, while paracrine hormones are produced in one cell type and affect an adjacent cell type. Neurohormones are similar to traditional hormones but differ only in their site of synthesis. Thus, neurohormones are produced in neural tissues and secreted into the bloodstream. Examples of these hormones are oxytocin and vasopressin, produced by the posterior pituitary gland, an extension of the CNS, and released into the bloodstream. In addition, neurohormones are produced by the hypothalamus at the base of the brain and are

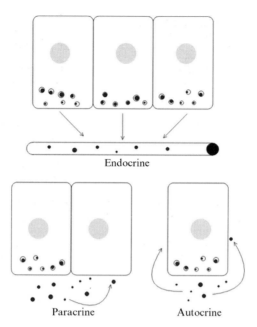

Fig. 3.1. Endocrine, paracrine and autocrine mechanisms of hormone delivery.

carried by a portal system to the anterior pituitary gland. These local, specialized hormones affect the anterior pituitary gland, inducing the stimulation or inhibition of anterior pituitary hormone secretion. Neurohormones must be distinguished from neurotransmitters, such as acetylcholine, serotonin and γ-aminobutyric acid (GABA), which provide communication across neural synapses. Neurotransmitters allow nerves to communicate with each other and with muscles.

Hormones regulate such diverse functions as respiration and metabolic rate, reproduction, cell, tissue and organ growth, glucose and mineral balance, blood pressure and gastric acid secretion. Table 3.1 illustrates the major endocrine glands and their hormones. This is not an all-inclusive compilation, as the focus is on hormones which are directly involved in growth. Hormones such as leptin, from adipose tissue, IGFs, from liver and many tissues, and vitamin D_3, synthesized by multiple tissues, are not included in this compilation of glands and hormones. Leptin, IGFs and vitamin D will be discussed thoroughly in subsequent chapters.

The location of the endocrine glands in the cow is shown in Fig. 3.2. The pituitary gland in the adult lies at the base of the brain, in a secure bony concavity of the skull called the sella turcica. The pituitary gland is attached to the brain and has three distinct portions, each synthesizing and secreting distinct hormones with far-ranging effects on growth and metabolism. Embryonically, the anterior pituitary gland (also called the pars distalis

Table 3.1. The endocrine glands and their hormones.

Gland	Hormones	Major actions
Anterior pituitary (pars distalis)	Growth hormone (GH) and somatotropin (ST)	Muscle/bone growth; protein synthesis; lipid and carbohydrate metabolism
	Adrenocorticotrophin (ACTH)	Controls adrenal cortex secretion of cortisol, corticosterone
	Thyrotrophin (thyroid-stimulating hormone (TSH))	Stimulates synthesis and release of thyroid hormones from thyroid
	Leutinizing hormone (LH) and follicle-stimulating hormone (FSH)	Regulate steroid synthesis and release from the gonads
Intermediate pituitary (pars intermedia)	Melanocyte-stimulating hormone (MSH)	Melanin synthesis in skin; skin darkening; appetite effects
Posterior pituitary (neurohypophysis)	Oxytocin	Milk ejection; uterine contraction
	Vasopressin, antidiuretic hormone (ADH)	Increases blood pressure; water reabsorption in kidney
Thyroid gland	Thyroxine (T_4), triiodothyronine (T_3)	Growth, neural development, regulates metabolic rate
	Calcitonin (CT)	Lowers blood calcium, phosphate
Parathyroid gland	Parathyroid hormone (PTH)	Increases blood calcium, lowers blood phosphate
Adrenal cortex	Cortisol, corticosterone	Induce gluconeogenesis, protein catabolism; anti-inflammatory actions
Adrenal medulla	Epinephrine (adrenalin)	Glycogen breakdown; increases blood glucose, blood flow, heart rate
	Norepinephrine (noradrenalin)	A neurotransmitter; increases blood pressure
Pancreatic islets (β-cells)	Insulin	Reduces blood glucose; increases tissue use of glucose, synthesis of lipid and protein
Pancreatic (α-cells)	Glucagon	Increases blood glucose; catabolism of protein, lipid; reduces gluconeogenesis
Testes	Testosterone	Male sexual characteristics, muscle growth
Ovaries, placenta	Oestrogens, progestagens (i.e. progesterone)	Female sexual characteristics; maintenance of pregnancy

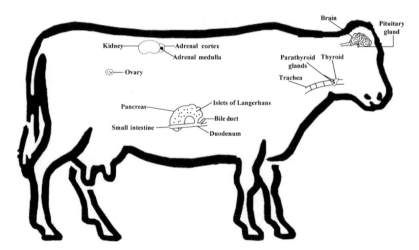

Fig. 3.2. Location of the endocrine glands in a cow.

or adenohypophysis) is derived from the ectoderm of the pharynx from an embryonic structure called Rathke's pouch. The anterior pituitary gland was once considered 'the master conductor of the endocrine orchestra', because it controls the function of many other endocrine glands such as the thyroid, adrenal cortex and the gonads. It is now known that each of the anterior pituitary hormones from the 'master conductor' is controlled by neurohormones secreted by the hypothalamus (discussed later) and the pars distalis might now be considered an 'assistant maestro'. In addition to the hormones which regulate other glands, the anterior pituitary produces GH, also called somatotropin (ST or STH), a hormone that plays an important role in growth and intermediary metabolism. The intermediate pituitary (pars intermedia), also a derivative of Rathke's pouch, lies between the anterior and posterior pituitary glands and secretes melanocyte-stimulating hormone (MSH) that has effects on skin pigmentation. The posterior pituitary, or neurohypophysis, has a separate embryonic derivation, and is formed by an evagination of the ventral diencephalon of the embryonic brain. It is a neural tissue and remains connected to the brain by the infundibular stalk. The posterior pituitary is the site of synthesis of oxytocin and vasopressin, neurohormones which regulate milk release and blood pressure.

The thyroid gland is a paired, butterfly-shaped organ which is located just below the larynx of the trachea. It secretes the hormones thyroxine (T_4) and triiodothyronine (T_3) which are essential for normal development of the CNS and play important roles in the regulation of metabolic rate and oxygen consumption by most cells of the body. The thyroid hormones are examples of hormones that are modified amino acids. As shown in Fig. 3.3, they are synthesized by iodination of tyrosine to form monoiodotyrosine and diiodotyrosine. These are then combined to form the active T_3 and T_4 thyroid hormones. The thyroid gland also secretes calcitonin (CT), a product of the C-cells of the thyroid. CT plays an important role in the growth and remodelling of bones,

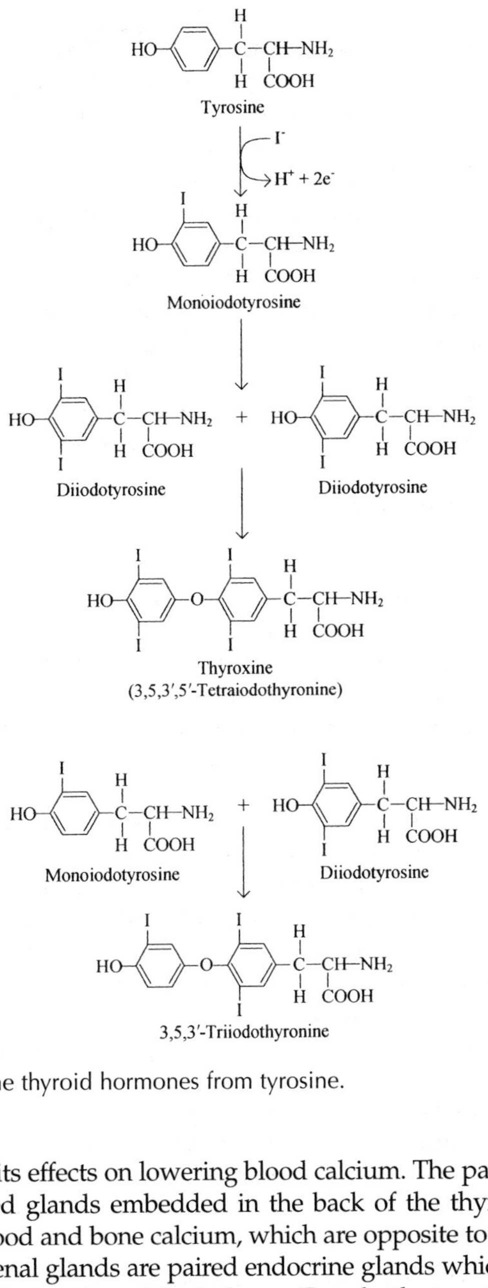

Fig. 3.3. Synthesis of the thyroid hormones from tyrosine.

reflected in its effects on lowering blood calcium. The parathyroid glands exist as two paired glands embedded in the back of the thyroid glands and have effects on blood and bone calcium, which are opposite to those of CT.

The adrenal glands are paired endocrine glands which reside on the anterior, or cephalic, portion of the kidneys. Grossly, the two functional areas of the adrenal glands are the outer cortex, which produces the corticosteroid hormones cortisol and corticosterone, and the inner medulla, which produces the catecholamines epinephrine (adrenaline) and norepinephrine (noradrenaline). Epinephrine is the primary circulating hormone produced by the adrenal medulla, while norepinephrine, which circulates in lower concentrations, acts primarily as a neurotransmitter. Adrenal hormones are released primarily in response to stress, and stimulate the mobilization of carbohydrates for use as energy by the body and by increasing heart rate, blood pressure and blood flow to skeletal muscle. These are the hormones which regulate the 'fight or flight' response, enabling an attacked animal to respond to a physical challenge with an appropriate response, either standing its ground and fighting or running away from danger. They also have important functions in the maintenance of daily physiological functions, such as providing a balance to the glucose-lowering effects of insulin. New approaches to the artificial regulation of body composition of meat animals utilize synthetic catecholamines (β-agonists), which take advantage of the lipolytic effects of these compounds to reduce carcass fat while increasing lean meat. These are discussed in detail in Chapter 10.

The pancreas produces the important glucose regulatory hormones insulin (from the β-cells of pancreatic islets) and glucagon, a product of pancreatic α-cells. Insulin is the hormone primarily responsible for stimulating the uptake and metabolism of glucose by most cells of the body, especially skeletal muscle and adipose tissue. Insulin is released in direct response to the increased blood glucose seen after a meal in non-ruminants. Levels of insulin in ruminants are less variable, as the rumen storage and release of energy sources (primarily volatile fatty acids (VFA)) is much slower and blood concentrations of glucose are not as variable as those seen in non-ruminants. The overall effect of insulin is to reduce blood glucose levels. The other major pancreatic hormone, glucagon, acts as an insulin counter-regulatory hormone, mobilizing glucose from hepatic stores and increasing blood glucose. Other hormones, which also have insulin counter-regulatory effects on blood glucose, include the corticosteroids and GH. All of these hormones act to mobilize glucose in one way or another with a resultant increase in blood glucose and a maintenance of blood glucose levels within a very narrow concentration range (4–7 mM in humans).

The gonads produce the sex-specific hormones oestrogen in females and testosterone in males. While these gonadal steroids play a natural role in the maintenance of sexual characteristics in their respective sexes in all animals, in ruminants they are also used as growth promotants, which increase feed efficiency and alter body composition. These are discussed in detail in Chapter 9.

In addition to classifying hormones based upon their source and function, they can also be described based upon chemical type or composition. This is important when the synthesis, use, mechanism of action and metabolism of different hormones are considered. There are three general chemical types of hormones.

1. *Protein/polypeptide* hormones consist of strings of amino acids. The pituitary gland produces only protein hormones, such as GH, adrenocorticotrophin (ACTH) and thyroid-stimulating hormone (TSH). Other glands, such as the pancreas, also produce relatively small polypeptide hormones such as insulin.

2. Some hormones are relatively simple *amino acid derivatives*, such as the thyroid hormones, which are derived from tyrosine, and the adrenal catecholamines epinephrine, norepinephrine and dopamine, also tyrosine derivatives.

3. *Steroids* are non-polar, lipid-soluble cholesterol derivatives. They are produced in the gonads, the adrenal glands and the placenta. Examples of these complex molecules include the sex steroids, oestrogens, progesterone and testosterone, and the adrenal steroids, cortisol and corticosterone.

Control of Pituitary Hormone Secretion

The release of hormones from the anterior pituitary is controlled by the hypothalamus, a specialized area of the midventral brain that lies beneath the third ventricle and thalamus of the brain and above the pituitary gland (Fig. 3.4). The hypothalamus consists of specialized neuronal cell bodies that synthesize and secrete releasing and inhibiting neurohormones into a capillary system called the hypophyseal portal system. This tiny specialized vascular system, which begins in a capillary bed in the hypothalamus and terminates in a capillary bed in the anterior pituitary, carries neurohormones from the hypothalamus to the anterior pituitary gland. The neuronal cell bodies in the hypothalamus are organized into specific areas called hypothalamic nuclei (Fig. 3.5). Each nucleus produces different releasing or inhibiting neurohormones that travel down axons to be released into the

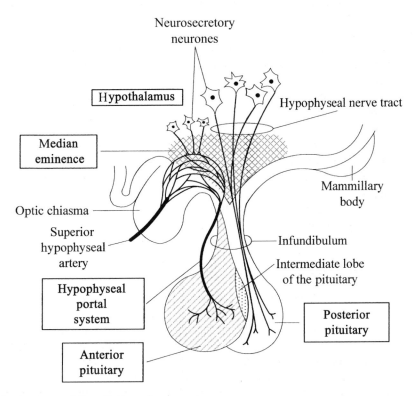

Fig. 3.4. Anatomy of the pituitary gland.

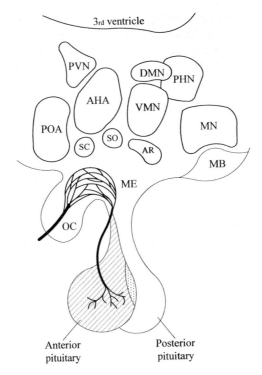

Fig. 3.5. Location of the hypothalamic nuclei. Abbreviations: AHA, anterior hypothalamic area; AR, arcuate nucleus; DMN, dorsomedial nucleus; MB, mammillary body; ME, median eminence; OC, optic chiasma; PHN, posterior hypothalamic nucleus; POA, preoptic area; PVN, paraventricular nucleus; SC, suprachiasmatic nucleus; SO, supraoptic nucleus; VMN, ventromedial nucleus.

hypophyseal portal system. For the most part, these are polypeptides containing anywhere from 10 to 43 amino acids. These neurohormones, also called hypophysiotropic hormones, stimulate or inhibit anterior pituitary hormone release (Table 3.2). The release of GH is under both positive and negative hypothalamic control. Growth hormone releasing hormone (GHRH) is a 43-amino acid polypeptide that stimulates GH release from

Table 3.2. Hypothalamic control of anterior pituitary hormone release.

Hormone	Hypothalamic neurohormones
GH	GHRH (+) and GHRIH (somatostatin) (−)
TSH	TRH (tripeptide)
LH/FSH	GnRH
PRL	Dopamine (−)
ACTH	CRF

the anterior pituitary, while growth hormone release-inhibiting hormone (GHRIH), or SS, a 14-amino acid polypeptide, inhibits GH release. Gonadotropin-releasing hormone (GnRH) is a 10-amino acid polypeptide that stimulates LH and FSH release, while thyrotropin-releasing hormone (TRH), a tripeptide, stimulates TSH release. The control of prolactin (PRL) secretion is under negative control by the neurotransmitter dopamine, a catecholamine derivative. The 41-amino acid corticotrophin-releasing hormone (CRH) stimulates ACTH release. The posterior, or neural, lobe of the pituitary is an extension of the CNS. Neural cell bodies in the hypothalamus synthesize the posterior pituitary hormones oxytocin and vasopressin. The axons of these neurones terminate in the posterior pituitary where they release these neurohormones into the systemic circulation.

Metabolic hormones such as insulin, GH and the adrenal catecholamines are involved in glucose, lipid and amino acid homeostasis. These hormones are controlled by nutritional intake and by systemic levels of metabolites, primarily glucose. Elevated levels of glucose also act on the hypothalamus and pituitary to reduce GH secretion while stimulating the release of insulin from the pancreas.

An essential aspect of the regulation of hormone concentrations involves a concept called 'negative feedback control'. This involves the self-regulation of hormone concentrations (Fig. 3.6). Thus, when blood hormone levels increase, this increase is detected by specific hormone receptors in the hypothalamus or the endocrine gland. When a hormone affects the gland that secretes it, this is called a short-loop negative feedback. A long-loop negative feedback arc is one that affects the control system preceding the gland of secretion. In this case, the hypothalamus, not the pituitary gland, would be affected. In response, the secretion of stimulatory neurohormones from the hypothalamus or the hormones themselves is reduced. This results in a reduction of hormone release from the gland and lower circulating levels of the hormone. These fine-tuned controls that regulate hormone concentrations ensure that hormone concentrations do not exceed a set point of concentration that would harm the animal.

As we have seen, the secretion of hormones from their glands and the regulation of hormone concentrations in the blood are mediated by internal control mechanisms acting within the body. It should be understood that interactions with external stimuli may also alter systemic hormone secretion. These mechanisms are especially important when dealing with environmental factors such as stress, photoperiod and temperature variation. Exteroceptive mechanisms that alter internal hormone secretion are mediated by the CNS. An external stimulus such as light from the environment can affect the endocrine system via photoreceptors in the eye, which, after transmission by the optic nerve to the brain, can be transmitted via nerve tracts to the hypothalamus where the hypothalamic output of releasing or inhibiting factors and pituitary hormones is altered. The release of pituitary hormones can alter thyroid or adrenal hormone release (Fig. 3.7). Other external factors such as stress and temperature changes affect the endocrine system in a similar manner, acting through external body receptors that relay messages to the brain and the hypothalamus, ultimately resulting in the increase or inhibition of hormone release.

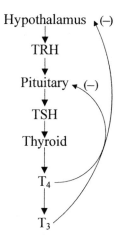

Hypothalamus ◢(−)

TRH

Pituitary ◤(−)

TSH

Thyroid

T_4

T_3

Fig. 3.6. Negative feedback loops of thyroid hormones on the hypothalamus and pituitary gland. Thyroid hormones act in a 'short-loop' at the level of the pituitary or a 'long-loop' at the level of the hypothalamus.

Hormone Receptors

Effects of hormones on target tissues are mediated by receptors located in the tissues affected by the respective hormones. Hormone receptors are cell proteins, which bind to and modulate hormone effects in target cells/tissues. They are highly specific for their hormone (ligand), are tissue-specific, present in very low concentrations in cells and have high affinity for hormones ($\sim 10^{-9}$–10^{-12} M). Receptors are the modulating molecules that confer tissue-specific actions on each hormone and mediate the cellular response to individual hormones. Receptors link the extracellular fluid environment of blood and extracellular matrix (ECM) with the interior of the cell. Binding of a hormone to its receptor sets in motion the sequence of stimulatory or inhibitory events within the targeted cell, which is characteristic of that cell's function as well as the effect of the hormone which impinges upon it.

There are two fundamental receptor types, those present in the plasma membrane of the cell and those which reside in the interior of the cell in the cytoplasm or nucleus. Plasma membrane receptors bind protein, polypeptide and amino acid-derived hormones. The plasma membrane receptors act as transducers, stimulating cytoplasmic second messengers which eventually affect gene expression in the nucleus of the target cell. Nuclear hormone receptors bind ligands within the cell, in the nucleus or cytoplasm. Typical ligands for intracellular receptors include small molecules that can easily pass through the plasma membrane, such as steroids, thyroid hormones and vitamin D. After binding their specific hormones, these receptors act directly on binding sites in the nucleus to alter gene expression. Thus, these hormone receptors are considered as ligand-activated transcription factors that regulate levels and rates of specific gene transcription.

Plasma membrane hormone receptors consist of three molecular domains: an extracellular domain that binds the hormonal ligand, a

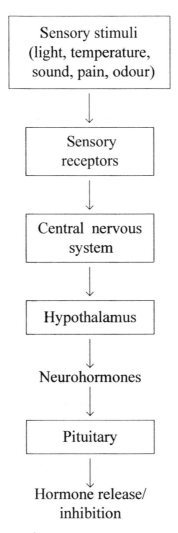

Fig. 3.7. Exteroceptive influence on hormone secretion.

lipophilic, transmembrane domain within the lipid bilayer and an intracellular cytoplasmic domain that activates intracellular signalling molecules.
These receptors can be classified into three types, based upon their structure,
associated kinases (enzymes that phosphorylate other proteins) and the second
messenger system activated by the receptor (Fig. 3.8). The intracellular domain
of the insulin and IGF-I receptors has an intrinsic tyrosine kinase (TK) activity,
which stimulates phosphorylation of the domain (autophosphorylation),
resulting in an active TK that, in turn, catalyses the phosphorylation of cytoplasmic substrates. This receptor is typical of insulin, IGF-I, epidermal growth
factor (EGF) and platelet-derived growth factor (PDGF). The second category of plasma membrane receptors is the cytokine receptors. Until they are
activated by hormone binding, cytokine receptors drift in the lipid bilayer as

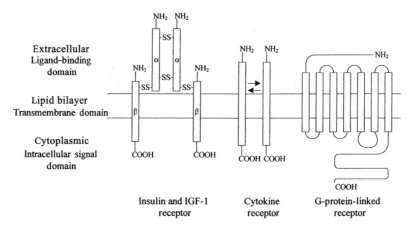

Fig. 3.8. Types of plasma membrane receptors.

single polypeptide monomers. Upon activation by hormone binding, these receptors associate with one another and form dimers. Dimerization activates cytoplasmic Janus kinase (JAK), a kinase that phosphorylates proteins on serine and threonine residues (a serine/threonine kinase). JAK binds to the receptor and phosphorylates it and activates cytoplasmic second messengers called signal transducers and activators of transcription (STATs). Cytokine receptors mediate the biological effects of GH, PRL, leptin and several interleukins. The last type of plasma membrane-associated receptors are called the seven transmembrane-domain receptors, or G-protein-linked receptors (GPLR). As the name implies, these receptors are snake-like proteins that wind in and out of the plasma membrane, with seven coils of the molecule passing through the membrane. These are ubiquitous receptors, which mediate the actions of many protein and amino acid-derived hormones, neurotransmitters and metabolites. Over 1000 of these receptors have been identified to date. Among the hormones which act through these receptors are TSH, parathyroid hormone (PTH), antidiuretic hormone (ADH), LH/FSH, calcitonin, ACTH and catecholamines.

Effector Molecules, Transducers and Second Messengers

The intracellular response systems for plasma membrane-bound hormone receptors function as 'relay systems' to convey a cell surface event (the binding of a hormone) to the interior of the cell, and eventually activate or silence specific genes in the nucleus. This is accomplished by a series of phosphorylations (catalysed by kinases) and dephosphorylations (by phosphatases) of cytoplasmic and nuclear proteins. All second messenger systems use phosphorylation/dephosphorylation events to increase or decrease enzyme activity, thus altering the intracellular message activity. What follows is a brief description of the cytoplasmic second messenger systems which mediate the effects of plasma membrane-bound receptors and their hormones.

The TK receptor family that binds insulin and IGF-I acts through two distinct pathways (Fig. 3.9). The first pathway is believed to mediate mitotic events. After tyrosine phosphorylation of the cytoplasmic protein, insulin receptor substrate-1 (IRS-1) by the receptor, the primary effector, mitogen-activated protein (MAP) kinase, alters gene expression and activates mitogenic pathways. The pathway that activates glucose uptake by the cell involves similar initial phosphorylations of cytoplasmic IRS-1 or IRS-2, but, in this case, the phophatidylinositol-3 (PI-3) kinase pathway is activated. This results in the movement of glucose transport molecules from sequestered intracellular sites to the plasma membrane.

The insulin and IGF-I receptors are very similar in structure, but have distinct hormone-binding specificities. The respective receptors have higher affinities, or binding strengths, for their specific molecules. Both insulin and IGF-I will bind to and activate the opposite receptor, but only at high concentrations. Thus, high levels of insulin can induce cell growth and mitosis via the MAP kinase pathway and high concentrations of IGF-I can induce the insulin-like effect of glucose transport via the PI-3 kinase pathway.

The GH/PRL receptor family consists of separate monomers which bind to ligands and associate with another receptor monomer to form an active receptor dimer (Fig. 3.10). Cytoplasmic JAK phosphorylates the receptor and, via phosphorylation, activates STAT to induce nuclear gene transcription. Alternatively, the activated receptor and JAK2 can stimulate the shc/Ras/MAP kinase pathway to induce gene expression and mitosis. Lastly, a minor pathway mediates transient insulin-like effects of GH on glucose transport into target cells via stimulation of the IRS/PI-3 kinase pathway.

The seven transmembrane-domain receptors, or GPLR, act through plasma membrane-bound G-proteins inside the cell which, in turn, activate other intracellular messengers. After ligand binding to the receptor, the receptor associates with and activates G-proteins. The G-proteins are bound

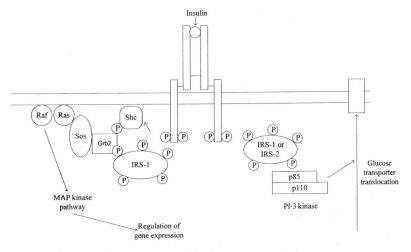

Fig. 3.9. Intracellular signalling pathways of the insulin and IGF-I receptor system.

to the cytoplasmic surface of the plasma membrane. They are guanidine triphosphatases (GTPases) that hydrolyse GTP to GDP, releasing phosphate.

The G-proteins are heterotrimeric molecules, consisting of three sub-units: α, β and γ. Functionally, there are only two subunits, the α subunit and (βγ) subunit, as the latter are tightly bound to one another. The α subunit of the G-proteins contains the nucleotide-binding site, which is inactive when GDP is bound to it. Contact with a hormone-activated receptor causes the release of GDP, which is immediately replaced with GTP. The GTP is rapidly hydrolysed to GDP. The active, GTP-bound form of the G-protein acts as a molecular switch that activates effector molecules such as adenylate cyclase (AC) and phospholipase-C (PLC) within the cell. As the GTP-bound form of the G-proteins is present only for a brief time, the activation of effector mol-ecules is rapid and transient.

The GPLR act through different effector molecules, depending upon the receptor, its ligand, the cell type and the G-linked protein. The G-proteins activate (or inhibit) AC or PLC. AC is bound to the cytoplasmic face of the plasma membrane and exists as ten isoforms. Activation of AC by G-proteins stimulates the formation of cyclic AMP (cAMP) from ATP. All receptors that act via cAMP use the stimulatory G-protein ($G_s\alpha$) of the α sub-unit to activate AC. Another α subunit isoform, the inhibitory G-protein ($G_i\alpha$), inhibits AC. Elevated intracellular concentrations of cAMP bind to and activate the enzyme protein kinase-A (PKA) (Fig. 3.11). PKA is a ser-ine/threonine kinase and alters the activities of other intracellular proteins

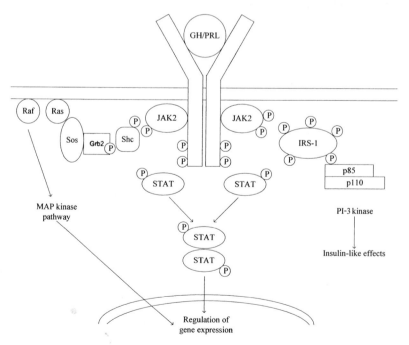

Fig. 3.10. Intracellular signalling pathways of the GH/PRL receptor.

by adding phosphates (from ATP) to their serine or threonine residues. The protein substrates for PKA are variable, and differ with cell type. In skeletal muscle, upon stimulation by epinephrine, PKA phosphorylates and activates enzymes involved in glycogen breakdown, while inactivating enzymes involved in glycogen synthesis. This results in a rapid increase in glucose availability. The phosphorylation of the cAMP regulatory-binding protein results in its activation, diffusion to the nucleus and binding to cAMP regulatory elements (CRE) of specific genes. In this way, hormonal stimulation of a cell alters the transcription of specific genes.

Activation of the plasma membrane-bound enzyme, PLC by GPLR provides an alternate pathway for the intracellular effects of hormones in specific tissues. Another isoform of the G-protein α subunit, the $G_q\alpha$ subunit, activates PLC. PLC exists as three forms: β, γ and δ and there are four isoforms of the β form (β_1–β_4). PLC-β mediates many of the effects of GPLR. PLC-β acts on a plasma membrane-bound inositol phospholipid, phosphatidylinositol (4,5)-bisphosphate (PIP$_2$), to form inositol 1,4,5-triphosphate (IP$_3$) and diacylglycerol (DAG) (Fig. 3.12). The products of this reaction, IP$_3$ and DAG, mediate separate intracellular processes. IP$_3$ diffuses through the cytoplasm to the SER. Here, it binds to an IP$_3$ receptor/calcium channel and stimulates Ca^{2+} influx into the cytoplasm from storage sites in the endoplasmic reticulum (Fig. 3.13). The elevated cytoplasmic concentrations of calcium bind to protein kinase-C (PKC) and stimulate its migration to the plasma membrane, where DAG remains bound. The most important role of DAG is to activate PKC, which in turn, phosphorylates additional cell-specific cytoplasmic proteins, resulting in their activation or repression.

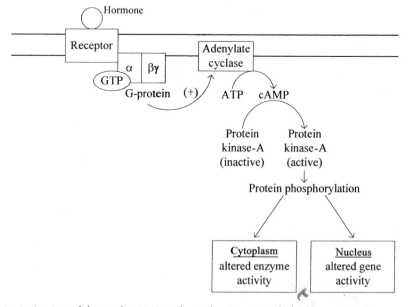

Fig. 3.11. Activation of the cyclic AMP pathway by G-protein-linked receptors.

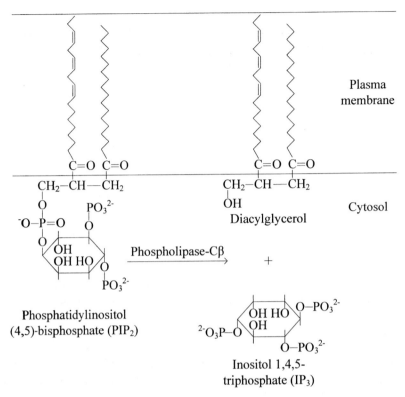

Fig. 3.12. Conversion of plasma membrane phosphatidylinositol (4,5)-bisphosphate to the intracellular messengers diacylglycerol and inositol 1,4,5-triphosphate.

The steroid hormone receptor family belongs to the superfamily of steroid/nuclear receptors, which are located in either the nucleus (thyroid hormones) or cytoplasm (glucocorticoids and sex steroids). These are ligand-activated nuclear transcription factors, which bind directly to promoter regions of specific genes in the nucleus. The steroid receptors consist of four functional domains which are responsible for hormone binding, nuclear localization, DNA binding and activation of transcription (Fig. 3.14). The glucocorticoid and oestrogen receptor molecules are transcription factors whose DNA-binding domain consists of 'zinc-fingers' (leucine-rich areas that contain zinc) that bind DNA and mediate the activity of these steroids on gene transcription.

There are four classes of the steroid/nuclear receptor superfamily. The first class of steroid receptors associate with one another to form homodimers, which bind to two palindromically arranged, hexanucleotide half sites on the gene promoter. The receptors for glucocorticoids, progesterone, oestrogen and androgens are members of this class. The second type of receptor, retinoid × receptors (R × R), forms heterodimers with unrelated steroid receptors and bind to direct repeat sites on the DNA promoter. The receptors for thyroid hormones and 1,25-dihydroxy vitamin D_3 belong to this class of steroid receptor. Dimorphic orphan receptors are so-called because their ligands are mostly

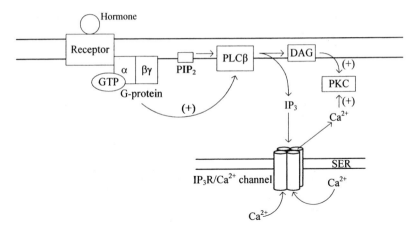

Fig. 3.13. Activation of the phosphoinositol pathway by G-linked protein receptors.

unknown. The last class of steroid receptors is called monomorphic orphan receptors, which have been noted, but whose ligands are unknown.

An overview of the actions of the endocrine system and hormones is given in Fig. 3.15, which outlines the pathways involved in the actions of protein and steroid hormones. This includes secretion from the endocrine glands into the bloodstream, transport via the systemic circulation, interaction with specific receptors in target cells and activation of intracellular

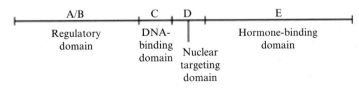

(A) Steroid receptor gene

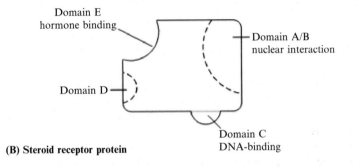

(B) Steroid receptor protein

Fig. 3.14. Steroid receptor gene and protein domains.

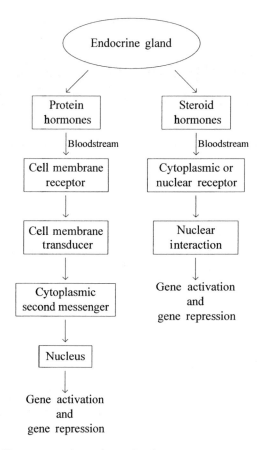

Fig. 3.15. Summary of hormone action – from gland to target DNA.

messenger systems and activation or repression of specific nuclear genes. The culmination of hormonal stimulation of a target cell results in the alteration of specific physiological processes in the target tissue.

References and Further Reading

Gomperts, B.D., Kramer, I.M. and Tatham, P.E.R. (2002) *Signal Transduction.* Academic Press, New York, 424 pp.

Hadley, M.E. (1984) *Endocrinology.* Prentice-Hall, Englewood Cliffs, New Jersey, 547 pp.

Pineda, M.H. and Dooley, M.P. (eds) (2003) *McDonald's Veterinary Endocrinology and Reproduction,* 5th edn. Iowa State Press, Blackwell, Ames, Iowa, 597 pp.

Squires, E.J. (2003) *Applied Animal Endocrinology.* CAB International, Wallingford, UK, 272 pp.

Starling, E.H. (1905) The chemical correlation of the functions of the body. *Lancet* ii, 339–341.

Turner, C.D. and Bagnara, J.T. (1976) *General Endocrinology,* 6th edn. W.B. Saunders, Philadelphia, Pennsylvania, 596 pp.

4 Development of Muscle, Skeletal System and Adipose Tissue

The focus of this book is on the hormonal regulation of the growth and development of the three tissues that are essential to the whole body development and composition of animals: muscle, bone and fat. The purpose of this chapter is to examine the normal growth and development of these three tissues. The effects of external agents, such as hormones, on the growth and metabolism of these tissues will be covered in subsequent chapters.

Embryonic Development and Cell Differentiation

As we have seen, development encompasses the alteration of body form. It also involves differentiation of cells into cells that assume specialized forms and functions, resulting in distinct tissues and organs which are capable of the processes we associate with animals. These differentiated cells have functions that range from gas exchange to reproduction, locomotion and consciousness.

The development of all animals begins with a single, undifferentiated cell, the diploid zygote (Fig. 4.1). The zygote results from the fertilization of a haploid oocyte by a haploid spermatozoon. This single cell will undergo mitosis within the zona pellucida, a gelatinous acellular layer surrounding the early oocyte and embryo. Cell replication results in a doubling of cell numbers with each round of mitosis. The replication of these undifferentiated cells forms of a ball of eight to 64 cells called a morula. The earliest differentiation of the embryo occurs when there are 128 to 256 cells, depending upon the animal species. At this time, a fluid-filled cavity, the blastocoele, forms and the embryo is called a blastocyst. The blastocyst is distinguished by two distinct groups of cells, the inner cell mass and the trophoblast. The inner cell mass contains cells destined to form the embryo proper and this cell aggregate is segregated to one side of the blastocoele. The trophoblast cells, surrounding the blastocoele, comprise the remainder of the blastocyst. The trophoblast will form the placenta and the embryonic membranes such as the amnion, chorion and allantois. After escape from the zona pellucida, the blastocyst attaches to the epithelium of the uterus and makes a physical connection to the maternal circulation via the placenta.

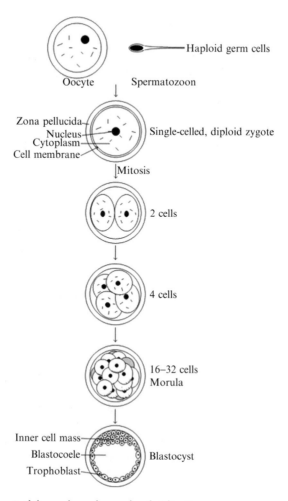

Fig. 4.1. Development of the early embryo after fertilization.

Traditionally, only the cells of the very early embryo, i.e. the first eight or 16 cells of the embryo, have been considered *totipotent*. In other words, only the undifferentiated, early embryonic cell was capable of forming a complete organism. In general, after cells had undergone differentiation, they were irreversibly altered and incapable of dedifferentiation into a more universal cell type capable of forming a functional organism. It is now known that most cells of the body, even in mature animals, under the proper conditions *in vitro*, can be induced to undergo dedifferentiation and are subsequently capable of forming entire living organisms through the process of cloning. *Pluripotent* cells or cell types, such as the mesoderm, are capable of limited formation of different tissues, and can differentiate into more than one cell type, such as muscle, bone or fat. They cannot form an entire organism.

After attachment to the uterus, embryonic cells multiply, migrate and differentiate to form three germ layers (Fig. 4.2), by a process called gas-

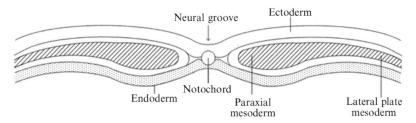

Fig. 4.2. Cross-section through an early developing embryo showing the three germ layers.

trulation. During embryonic development, the three germ layers differentiate into the specific organs and tissues of the animal. The outermost of these layers is called the ectoderm and it will form the brain, spinal cord and skin of the animal. The inner layer is called the endoderm and it will form many of the internal organs of the animal, including most of the gastrointestinal system. The middle layer of cells in the embryos is called the mesoderm, and it is this layer which gives rise to three tissues that are the primary focus of this book, bone, muscle and fat, as well as cartilage, blood, dermis and connective tissues such as tendons, ligaments and joint capsules.

The paraxial mesoderm, lying on either side of the embryonic neural tube, is a specialized type of mesodermal tissue which forms the embryonic somites (Figs. 4.3 and 4.4). The somites consist of segmented blocks of cell condensations which form sequentially along both sides of the embryonic neural tube (future spinal cord) and notochord (an embryonic support structure beneath the neural tube) during embryogenesis. The somites form sequentially in an anterior to posterior (head-to-tail) sequence, with the somites closest to the head forming first. Different areas of the somites will differentiate into different structures of the body. The ventral portion of the somite is called the sclerotome. It will differentiate into the bones of ribs and vertebrae. The rest of the somite, called the dermomyotome, is divided into three developmental regions. The dorsal dermomyotome will form some skeletal muscles and the dermal skin of the trunk. The epaxial dermomyotome will form the epaxial musculature of the back. The ventrolateral portion of the somite will give rise to the hypaxial musculature of the trunk and limbs. When muscle formation is initiated, the progenitor muscle cells of the somites (myoblasts) detach from the body of the somite and migrate to specific areas of muscle formation, such as the embryonic limb buds.

Another type of mesoderm is called the mesenchyme, a type of loosely packed aggregation of mesodermal cells (mesenchymal cells), suspended in the gelatinous ECM located between the ectodermal and endodermal germ layers. These cells are motile, in some cases contain migrating cells from the somites. Mesenchymal cells migrate through the body to form many of the skeletal, connective tissue, blood and smooth muscle systems. Another type of important cell derived from mesoderm is the fibroblast. These cells are widely distributed in the embryo and the adult. Fibroblasts form connective

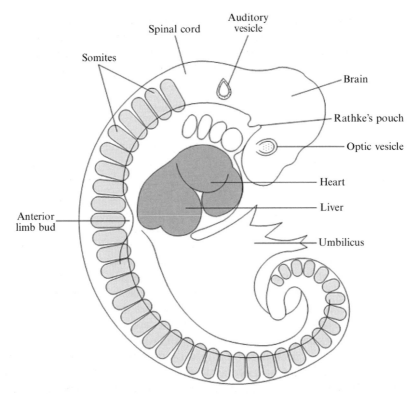

Fig. 4.3. Diagram of a 5 mm pig embryo showing relationships between somites, anterior limb bud and spinal cord.

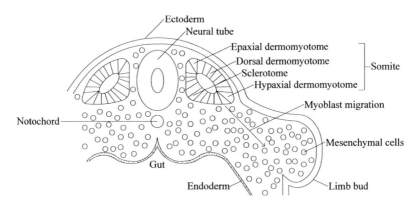

Fig. 4.4. Cross-section through an embryo showing the somites at the levels of the limb bud.

tissue cells that produce and secrete the ECM. They are involved in the growth, wound repair and accessory physiological processes of all tissues. They are relatively undifferentiated cells and, under appropriate conditions, are capable of differentiating into osteoblasts and chondroblasts in the adult.

Cell Proliferation and Differentiation

Differentiation of cells involves the assumption of a specialized function. For example, differentiated cells may be capable of contraction (of muscles), lipid storage (adipose) or the propagation of a nerve impulse, the formation of an idea. These functions are accompanied by the expression of specific genes for specific products related to cell function such as the genes for contractile proteins in muscle or lipogenic genes in adipose tissue. Cellular differentiation follows a generalized pattern (Fig. 4.5), which is applicable to all tissues. An undifferentiated cell undergoes a round of mitotic proliferation, which results in two daughter cells. One of these cells, in turn, is committed to undergo differentiation in which the cell assumes an essentially irreversible specialized function. Accordingly, in many cases, the second daughter cell remains undifferentiated, and becomes mitotically quiescent. This reserve stem cell provides a reservoir of cells, which can be activated under appropriate conditions when additional differentiated cells are required. The sequence of mitotic proliferation followed by differentiation is generally, although not always, a mutually exclusive event. Proliferating cells are devoting their metabolic energy and genetic resources towards increasing cell numbers. It is only upon appropriate stimuli that these cells alter their functions, cease cell division and begin the processes associated with differentiation.

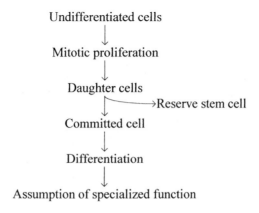

Fig. 4.5. General pattern of cell differentiation.

The Skeletal System and Bone Growth

The importance of bone tissue to animal agriculture is illustrated by the costly problems associated with bone dysfunction. Recent changes in the genetics and nutrition of livestock animals have led to increased growth rates, mature animal sizes and weights. Associated with these fundamental alterations of animal metabolism and physiology is an increased incidence of long bone anomalies. Modern domesticated animals are beset with an array of skeletal anomalies associated with their intense selection for rapid growth. For example, half of the broiler chickens in the USA are affected by tibial dyschondroplasia, in which growth plate cartilage accumulates in the tibia and femur, leading to lameness and increased leg fractures. A similar problem in swine, osteochondrosis, is characterized by a lack of bone formation (ossification) in the growth plate of the load-bearing bones. These problems lead to losses of millions of dollars to the livestock industry and it is important to understand the growth and development of the important, yet often overlooked, skeletal system. Traditionally, a great deal of attention has been paid to the obvious components of body composition in farm animals, the skeletal muscle and fat. The increased body size, altered composition and rapid growth rates of modern farm animals require a reordering of our priorities. A basic knowledge of bone growth and development, and its regulation, are essential for the optimal management and successful production of food animals.

Bone is a dynamic, living tissue which has several functions that are important to the metabolism, growth and normal functions of animals. Most obviously, bone provides a structural support for the body, providing attachment points for muscles to allow for body movements. The high strength to weight ratio of bone is essential to provide mobility for the animal. Of course, bone must also be flexible, providing some elasticity to the movements of animals. Bone also has important metabolic functions that are important for whole body homeostasis. It provides a reservoir for several minerals including calcium, phosphate, magnesium, sodium and carbonate in the body. These minerals are in equilibrium with blood minerals and are mobilized from or deposited in the bone matrix depending upon the physiological requirements of that animal. Another essential function of bone is the production of blood cells by bone marrow. Marrow is also the site of production of stem cell precursors that will form osteoblasts and osteoclasts of bone. Recent observations suggest that bone marrow may also be the source of stem cells for other tissues, such as skeletal muscle and adipose tissue. Thus, bone plays important roles in several vital processes associated with the animal's well-being. Bone has not only a purely mechanical and structural role, but also plays essential physiological roles in the maintenance of electrolyte homeostasis and the production of stem cells. Like cartilage, bone is a highly specialized type of connective tissue. The ECM of bone consists primarily of mineralized crystalline deposits of calcium and phosphate, and forms the majority of the bone mass. This extensive ECM surrounds the relatively sparse bone cells embedded in this rigid matrix.

Types of Bones and Gross Anatomy

There are two types of bone, based on their embryonic origins. Membranous bone (also called intramembranous bone) is formed *de novo* from bone cells. Examples of membranous bone are the flat bones of the skull, i.e. the calvarium, or skullcap of the head. Calvarial osteoblasts are derived directly from precursor mesenchymal stem cells. The second type of bone is cancellous bone. Most bones, including those of the appendages, are cancellous bones. Also called endochondral bone, this type of bone is formed by replacing an existing cartilage model with bone. This model is formed when embryonic mesenchymal cells proliferate, undergo hypertrophy and form condensations of cells at the site of future bone formation. The mesenchymal cells differentiate into chondroblasts that deposit the ECM of cartilage, forming a miniature cartilaginous model of the future bone. When completely surrounded by matrix, they are then called chondrocytes. Chondrocytes proliferate, differentiate and hypertrophy and secrete a cartilage matrix that is mineralized.

The long cancellous bones of the skeleton have a characteristic gross anatomy which relates to the function of these bones (Fig. 4.6). This includes the central shaft, which is called the *diaphysis* (pl. diaphyses). Long bone ossification in the embryo begins in the central region of the diaphysis where ossification of cartilage first occurs. The inner layer of the long bone, which surrounds the marrow, is called the endosteum. Osteoblasts and osteoclasts responsible for growth and remodelling of the bone are found here. The outer layer of the long bone, the periosteum, contains osteoblasts, osteocytes and fibroblasts. This is where the increase in bone diameter occurs. The end of the bones is called the *epiphysis* (pl. epiphyses). This is the secondary centre of ossification, where long bone mineralization continues in the embryo. The *epiphyseal plate*, or *growth plate*, is the strip of cartilage between the epiphysis and the diaphysis. The epiphyseal plate contains chondroblasts and chondrocytes, which form the cartilage template for linear bone growth. The portion of the long bone between the diaphysis and the epiphysis is called the *metaphysis*. This is where bone mineralization of the cartilage matrix occurs. The epiphyseal plate is generally fused (ossified) around the time of puberty when linear growth ceases.

Bone Cells and Bone Matrix Formation

Bone consists of three major types of cells with different functions: osteoblasts, osteoclasts and osteocytes. Osteoblasts are derived from mesenchymal cells during embryonic development and from mesenchymal stem cells in the periosteum or stromal stem cells in the marrow (endosteum) after bone formation. The precursor cells become committed to the osteoblast cell lineage, proliferate and differentiate into preosteoblasts. Preosteoblasts are committed to differentiate into osteoblasts. Osteoblasts are precursors of mature osteocytes. Osteoblasts are fully differentiated cells that are responsible for the

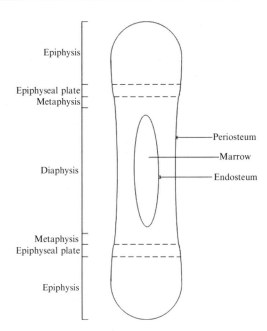

Epiphysis

Epiphyseal plate
Metaphysis

Diaphysis

Periosteum

Marrow

Endosteum

Metaphysis
Epiphyseal plate

Epiphysis

Fig. 4.6. Anatomy of a long bone.

production of bone matrix. Osteoblasts display a cell phenotype which is typical of a protein-producing cell. They contain extensive RER and a well-developed Golgi apparatus. The primary function of the osteoblasts is to secrete the organic ECM, or osteoid. Initially, the osteoid is not mineralized but serves as a template for mineralization. In addition to secretion of collagen, the osteoblasts are also the source of extracellular collagenase. Collagenase is secreted during bone remodelling to degrade the collagen portion of the organic matrix. Collagenases exist in three isoforms (collagenase 1, 2 and 3), all of which degrade Type I collagen in the matrix with similar efficiencies. Secretion of collagenases is stimulated or inhibited during different developmental stages and during bone remodelling and repair.

The organic matrix of bone consists primarily of Type I collagen (90–95%) with the remainder composed of other proteins and proteoglycans. Proteoglycans are large molecular complexes consisting of 95% carbohydrates and 5% proteins. Along with collagen, many minor proteins and glycoproteins are secreted by osteoblasts into the osteoid. These include proteoglycans such as decorin and biglycan. Both bind to chondroitin or dermatin sulphate. Decorin binds to (decorates) collagen fibrils while biglycan occupies the pericellular area of osteoblasts and osteocytes. Transforming growth factor-β (TGF-β) binds to both of these molecules. Decorin and biglycan are believed to act as matrix organizers, helping to orient the collagen molecules. Other matrix proteins contain the arginine, glycine, aspartic acid (RGD) sequences that bind to cell surface integrin receptors to provide matrix–cell interactions and adhesion. These include fibronectin and thrombospondin. The PDGF growth factors also bind to thrombospondin and osteonectin. Another matrix protein, osteonectin, binds calcium, hydroxyapatite and several collagen isoforms (I, II and IV). Osteonectin is thought to act as an anti-adhesive component, reducing cell adhesion to the matrix and altering cell morphology. Osteopontin is a glycoprotein that contains the RGD sequence for integrin binding. It is secreted by osteoblasts that are nearing maturity. Its deposition leads to the first mineralization of the matrix and thus, serves as a marker for osteoblast maturation and bone mineralization.

Osteoblasts also secrete hyaluronic acid, a large carbohydrate that forms a portion of the ECM. It consists of a repeating disaccharide of glucuronic acid and N-acetylglucosamine. It is often found in association with multiple core proteins that bind to the long axis of hyaluronic acid, forming a bottle-brush structure. As with many carbohydrates found in proteoglycans, hyaluronic acid contains acetylated amino sugars. For this reason these carbohydrates are called glycosaminoglycans. Hyaluronic acid and other glycosaminoglycans are able to bind water up to 10,000 times their own volume to yield gels and thus, to capture space for further matrix deposition. Other glycosaminoglycans include the chondroitin sulphates, polymers of glucuronic and N-acetyl sugars and keratin sulphate, a sulphur-rich minor protein component.

During the development of the osteoblast, there is a distinct sequence of events that characterize its differentiation. In the early stages, osteoblasts undergo cell mitosis and proliferation. The first components of osteoid secreted by the osteoblasts are Type I collagen and fibronectin. As the cell continues to mature, they continue to secrete collagen and begin to produce alkaline phosphatase. Alkaline phosphatase is an enzyme complex that is often used as a molecular marker for osteoblast differentiation. Alkaline phosphatase hydrolyses pyrophosphate and ATP, both inhibitors of matrix calcification. This allows the initial formation of hydroxyapatite crystals on the osteoid. Later in the life cycle of the osteoblast, collagen production slows and osteocalcin and osteopontin are secreted.

The mineralization of the organic matrix to form the rigid structure we know as bone is regulated by osteoblasts, although the mechanisms are not completely understood. High local concentrations of Ca^{2+} and PO_4^{3-} are required for the formation of calcium phosphate precipitates. Mature osteoblasts secrete membrane-bound matrix vesicles that bud from cytoplasmic processes of these cells. These vesicles are rich in alkaline phosphatase and allow the precipitation of calcium phosphate and the crystallization of hydroxyapatite molecules [$Ca_{10}(PO_4)_6(OH)_2$] on to the organic matrix. Collagen serves as a template for mineral deposition and may regulate the process of mineralization. The inorganic, insoluble hydroxyapatite forms the mature bone shape and function.

After osteoblasts are completely surrounded by mineralized matrix, they differentiate into osteocytes. The osteocytes are thought to be responsible for the maintenance of the bone. Osteocytes continue to produce matrix proteins and are capable of limited bone resorption. Osteocytes reside in pockets in the bone called osteocytic lacunae, surrounded by the mineralized

ECM of the bone (Fig. 4.7). Deposition of mineral makes the matrix imper-
meable and specialized channels in the bony matrix, called canaliculi, allow
osteocytes to physically connect each other. Osteocytes fill the canaliculi
with long cytoplasmic projections, which form gap junctions with adjacent
osteocytes. These specialized connections allow intercellular communication
between the osteocytes. The canaliculi and the lacunae contain an extracellular fluid space between the plasma membrane and the bone matrix. This
fluid, which moves throughout the network of osteocytes, is the only source
of nutrients for the osteocyte.

Osteoclasts and bone resorption

Osteoclasts are specialized bone cells responsible for the resorption of mineralized bone. These cells are large, multinucleated phagocytes, containing
four to 29 nuclei. Osteoclasts are derived from the fusion of circulating
mononucleated blood cells (monocytes) derived from the bone marrow.
They reside on the surfaces of the bone, primarily in the marrow and periosteum, and play an essential role in bone resorption that is required for
growth, remodelling and fracture repair of bones. Osteoclasts are characterized by an abundance of mitochondria, Golgi apparati and lysosomes.

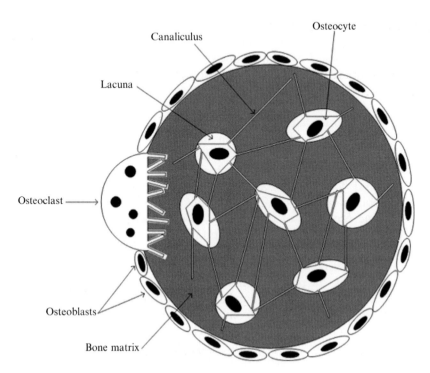

Fig. 4.7. Relationship of the primary bone cells.

The most conspicuous characteristic of the osteoclasts relates to their bone-resorbing function (Fig. 4.8). The plasma membrane of osteoclasts contains multiple, deep folds on the cell side that faces the bone surface called a ruffled border. Osteoclasts are tethered to the bone surface by an encircling zone of attachment called the sealing zone. The sealing zone acts to attach the osteoclast to the bone matrix and to isolate the underside of the osteoclast from the external environment. The sealing zone attachment occurs via integrin receptors on the osteoclast plasma membrane that bind to RGD sequences in matrix proteins. This forms a bone-resorbing compartment beneath the osteoclast where bone matrix can be degraded. Bone resorption by osteoclasts occurs by acidification and solubilization of hydroxyapatite crystals and by proteolysis of matrix proteins within the sealing zone. The osteoclast produces H^+ via the action of carbonic anhydrase within the cell. The protons are pumped across the ruffled border membrane by proton pumps, reducing the pH of the sealing zone. The osteoclast also secretes a variety of lysosomal and non-lysosomal proteases into the bone-resorbing compartment to degrade the matrix. Lysosomes provide the protease, cathepsin K and acid phosphatase. Non-lysosomal proteases include the matrix metalloproteinases, collagenase and gelatinase B. This combination of enzymes and protons acts to dissolve the bone matrix and results in small 'craters' on the surface of the bone, which can be remodelled or replaced with new matrix.

Regulation of osteoclast function

The activities of osteoclasts are regulated by osteoblasts. Receptors for most external factors, such as hormones and growth factors that induce bone

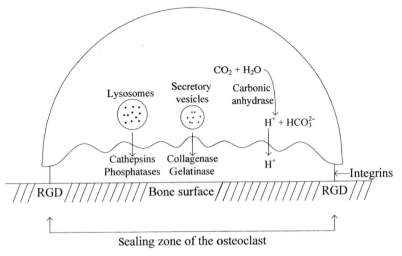

Fig. 4.8. Components of osteoclast attachment and bone dissolution.

resorption, are found in osteoblasts, not osteoclasts. Osteoblasts also produce growth factors and cytokines that influence the differentiation and function of osteoclasts, either by direct paracrine actions or after deposition into the matrix. The effects of osteoblasts on osteoclast differentiation and function are mediated by a recently discovered receptor–ligand system, called the RANK/RANKL system (Fig. 4.9). This system is composed of three components. The membrane-bound receptor activator of NFκB (RANK) receptor, a member of the tumour necrosis factor (TNF) receptor family, is present in osteoclast progenitor cell plasma membrane. The plasma membrane of osteoblasts contains the immobilized RANK transmembrane ligand (RANKL) that binds to and activates the RANK receptor molecule when osteoblasts and osteoclast precursor cells are in contact with one another. In addition, osteoblasts secrete a soluble decoy receptor called osteoprotegerin (OPG) that binds to and inactivates RANKL. NFκB is the cytoplasmic mediator of RANK receptor in osteoclasts. Cell-to-cell contact between osteoblast and presumptive or mature osteoclasts allows binding and activation of the

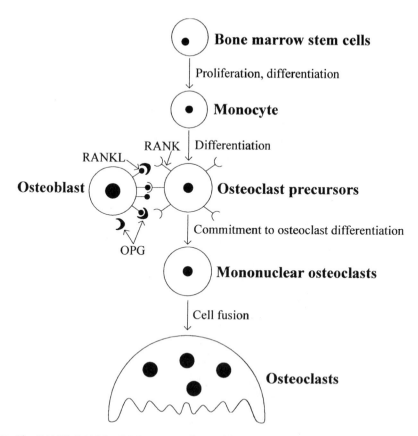

Fig. 4.9. The RANK, RANKL, OPG system of osteoblasts and osteoclasts.

RANK/RANKL system. This induces the differentiation and activation of osteoclasts and bone resorption. The negative regulation of osteoclast formation occurs by osteoblastic secretion of OPG. OPG acts as a decoy receptor, binding RANKL and inhibiting its binding to RANK, reducing the differentiation of osteoclasts. As a result of RANK/RANKL interaction, formation of osteoclasts and thus, bone resorption is enhanced.

The Epiphyseal Plate

The anatomy of the epiphyseal plate and the relationships of the cells involved in long bone growth are shown in Fig. 4.10. Chondrocytes are arranged in columns that are maintained by mineralization of the spaces between the columns. Mineralization of the cartilaginous matrix begins in the zone of proliferating chondrocytes, farthest from the growth plate, and becomes denser around the hypertrophic chondrocytes. Some mineralized cartilage is resorbed at the marrow cavity margins by osteoclasts to provide room for new bone deposition and vascular growth. The remaining mineralized cartilage provides the surface for osteoblasts to differentiate and mineralize the ECM of bone.

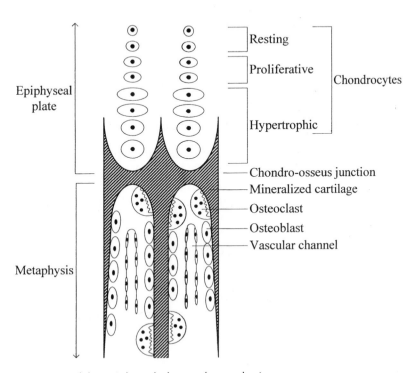

Fig. 4.10. Anatomy of the epiphyseal plate and metaphysis.

Skeletal Muscle Development

Along with the skeletal system, skeletal muscle provides the animal with the physical support to remain upright and the locomotory skills to move, run and feed. The diaphragm is also composed of skeletal muscle, and thus, skeletal muscle is essential for the regulation of respiration in the animal. Muscle is, of course, the primary product of meat animal production, forming the basis for an extensive animal agriculture production system and one of the primary sources of dietary protein in many cultures. In many animals, the majority of skeletal muscle development occurs during embryonic development. This provides the newborn animal with immediate mobility, allowing it to accompany adults and to avoid predation. Many farm animals 'hit the ground running' and are capable of standing, nursing and walking immediately after birth.

Skeletal muscle is a tissue that is specialized to provide contraction forces for movement. Mature skeletal muscle is unique in that it is composed of multinucleated, non-mitotic cells containing large quantities of large, insoluble proteins that provide muscle strength, elasticity and contraction. Muscles function in conjunction with the nervous system, which provides the stimulus for muscle contraction. Muscle is also dependent upon its interaction with the skeletal system, which provides the framework for muscle attachment and the support for muscle movement and, subsequently, together the skeleton and the skeletal muscle aid in the maintenance of body form and shape. Compared to the skeletal system, the nomenclature and interaction of the cells involved in skeletal muscle formation are relatively straightforward.

Embryonic formation of skeletal muscle

Skeletal muscle of the body and limbs is derived from mesodermal cells which differentiate into the muscle progenitor cells, the myoblasts. Myoblasts are mononucleated cells, which are capable of mitosis and fusion with other myoblasts to form multinucleated cells. Myoblasts accumulate small amounts of the myofibrillar proteins actin and myosin during maturation, but myoblasts are not contractile cells. Myoblasts fuse with one another to form the embryonic myotubes, characterized by the presence of multiple, centrally located nuclei within each cell. A single myotube may contain hundreds of nuclei. After fusion of myoblasts to form myotubes, the synthesis of myofibrillar proteins is accelerated. The mature differentiated muscle cell is called a muscle fibre or a myofibre. Myofibres are characterized by additional actin and myosin accumulation, an increase in cell size and the migration of cell nuclei to a peripheral location, making room for the accumulating contractile apparatus of the myofibre.

In vertebrate animals, mesodermal somites of the embryo give rise to the muscles of the limbs and body, while local condensations of mesodermal cells form the skeletal muscle of the head. As described earlier, the somites are paired condensations of mesoderm that form along both sides of the embryonic spinal column. The hypaxial musculature of the limbs and body wall is derived from the myogenic precursor cells residing in the lateral portion of the somites. The epaxial musculature of the back and intercostal (rib) muscles is derived from the medial halves of the somites. Embryonic limb muscle myogenesis begins shortly after the formation of the three primary germ layers (a process termed gastrulation), in the first third of gestation, when myogenic progenitor cells in the somites adjacent to the limb buds cells delaminate, or detach from the somites. This is followed by the migration of these cells to the sites of muscle formation, for example, the embryonic limb buds. In the limb buds, myoblasts form dorsal and ventral aggregates of cells surrounding the cartilage primordia that will later form endochondral bone. Genes that regulate muscle formation are activated and the myoblasts begin to actively proliferate. This ensures that there is an adequate population of myoblast progenitors capable of fusing to form mature, functional skeletal muscle. Myoblast proliferation is followed by cessation of mitosis and differentiation into myotubes. In this process, myoblasts fuse with one another to form multinucleated myotubes that synthesize large amounts of the contractile proteins (Fig. 4.11). Embryonic myoblasts fuse with one another to form primary myotubes, which defines the type, shape and location of muscles in the adult. During the second third of gestation, *fetal* myoblasts form secondary myotubes, which form around the primary myotubes. The secondary myotubes undergo hypertrophy and attach to other myotubes via tight connections called gap junctions, allowing cell-to-cell communication between the myotubes. The fetal myoblast period, when secondary muscle fibres are formed, determines the ultimate number of fibres in the adult. Myofibre formation is generally completed during the first two-thirds of prenatal development, although this process is species-dependent.

Skeletal muscle satellite cells

Skeletal muscle is capable of limited repair and regeneration and grows throughout adulthood. Both muscle DNA content and muscle mass increase during the postnatal period. It is estimated that 70% to more than 90% of myofibre DNA accumulates postnatally. This occurs despite the observations that myofibre numbers are fixed at birth and myofibres are incapable of mitosis. As mature myofibres are incapable of mitosis, the mechanism of postnatal myofibre DNA accumulation was unknown until relatively recently. In the 1960s, muscle satellite cells were discovered. Satellite cells are considered the adult equivalent of embryonic myoblasts and provide new nuclei to growing or damaged skeletal muscle fibres. These cells lie just outside the cell membrane of the mature myofibre, between the cell and underlying the basement membrane. These tiny, mononucleated cells consist almost entirely of nuclei, with very little cytoplasm. Only a few satellite cells are present in muscle. It has been estimated that satellite cells account for 1%

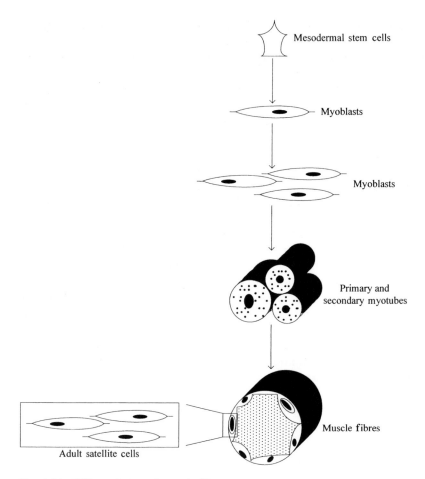

Fig. 4.11. Differentiation of muscle fibres.

to 10% of the nuclei present in muscle fibres. Upon activation, satellite cells proliferate, fuse with each other and with the myofibre sarcolemma and add more nuclei to the myofibre. Some of the satellite cells resulting from replication return to quiescence and retain their extracellular site to assure that the pool of progenitor cells is not depleted. Fusion of satellite cells with mature muscle fibres results in an increase in adult muscle DNA content that can support an increased muscle mass. In the large, multinucleated muscle fibre, it is thought that a nucleus has only a limited sphere of influence and can affect only the cytoplasm immediately around it. As the myofibres are enormous cells, spanning up to 100 μm in length, multiple nuclei are required to provide the synthetic machinery needed to increase muscle protein synthesis that must accompany cell growth. Fusion of satellite cells with adult muscle fibres provides a mechanism to increase the DNA content of the non-mitotic muscle cell, without nuclear replication.

Satellite cells and myoblasts share many things in common. Both are myogenic cell precursors that can undergo mitosis and fusion to form the multinucleated myofibres and it has been suggested that satellite cells are simply adult myoblasts. There are several lines of evidence that myoblasts and satellite cells are distinct from one another and are not simply different developmental stages of the same cells. The most obvious difference between these cell types is, of course, developmental. Satellite cells are post-natal stem cells, while myoblasts are present during embryonic and fetal development. In contrast, it has been shown that myotubes derived from satellite cells contain ~1/3 of the actin per myotube nucleus than myoblast-derived myotubes. Tumour-promoting phorbol esters have different effects on these cells. They block myoblast differentiation, but do not affect the differentiation of satellite cells. Acetylcholine receptor channels are present in satellite cells but are seen only after differentiation in myoblasts. In addition, myoblasts are active in DNA synthesis and mitosis, while satellite cells are primarily quiescent cells that undergo mitosis only upon activation. Finally, satellite cells are much smaller than myoblasts. Thus, satellite cells appear to be a separate population of adult stem cells, which are morphologically and functionally distinct from fetal and embryonic myoblasts. Satellite cells are derived from adult muscles and used in primary cultures to study muscle growth and differentiation. A number of immortalized myoblast cell lines are used as experimental models to study myogenesis. Examples of these include the L6, C2C12 and C2 myoblast cell lines.

Myofilaments, Myofibrils and Sarcomeres

Mature muscle cells are composed of contractile proteins arranged into functional contractile units called myofibrils. Myofibrillar proteins account for the majority of proteins in the muscle cell, comprising 55% to 65% of the total protein in a myofibre. Myofibrils are long threads of protein composed of multiple repeating sarcomeres, connected end-to-end. Myofibrils are massive bundles of myofilaments, about 1 to 2 μm in diameter and extending the length of the muscle fibre, up to several millimetres. There are thousands of myofibrils in each muscle cell, arranged side-by-side and connected to each other with proteins called intermediate filaments. The intermediate filaments provide physical support for the myofibrils and join the myofibrils into a single cohesive unit that provides a unified contraction force. A major intermediate filament, often used as a marker for skeletal muscle, is the protein desmin. Sarcomeres are the functional contractile unit of the muscle and are made up of the two major myofilament proteins, actin and myosin. Actin and myosin generate the contraction forces within the sarcomere. Alteration of the thick myosin filaments with the thin actin filaments within the sarcomere give the skeletal muscle its typical striated, or striped, appearance. The anatomy of a sarcomere, at rest and during muscle contraction, is shown

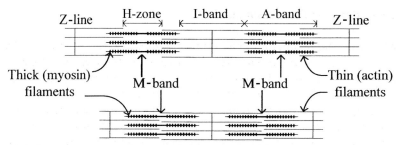

(A) Two sarcomeres, at rest, above, and after contraction, below

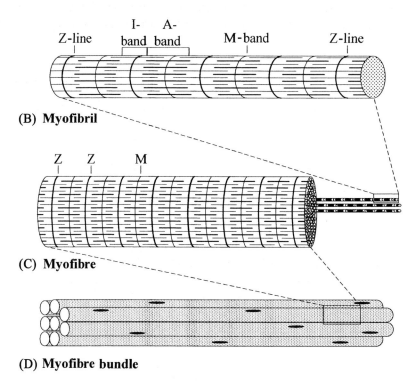

(B) Myofibril

(C) Myofibre

(D) Myofibre bundle

Fig. 4.12. The organization of sarcomeres into myofibrils and myofibres.

in Fig. 4.12. The entire sarcomere extends from Z-line to Z-line. The region occupying the outer portions of the sarcomere, near the Z-lines, is composed solely of the actin molecule and is called the I-band. The central portion of the sarcomere contains the myosin molecule and is called the A-band. The portion of the A-band that contains only myosin is called the H-zone. The dark centre of the H-zone is known as the M-band and it consists solely of the dense, central portion of the myosin molecule.

Sarcomeric proteins: actin, myosin and titin

Myosin is the most abundant protein in muscle cells. It forms the thick filament of the sarcomere. The myosin molecule (~220 kDa) is a dimer that consists of a long, rod-like tail composed of two intertwining heavy myosin
molecules that form an α helix, and a globular head (Fig. 4.13). Two myosin
light chains, which have regulatory functions, are associated with the neck
region of the heavy myosin chains. The myosin tail provides an anchor that
maintains the position of the myosin heavy chain (MHC). The myosin tail is
attached to the globular head domain of myosin via a hinged neck region.
The neck region allows the head of the myosin chain to 'contract', or
flex, much like your wrist allows your hand to flex, moving up and down

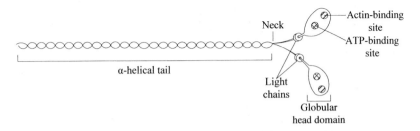

(A) Myosin

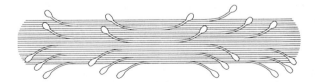

(B) Sarcomeric bundle of myosin molecules (thick filament)

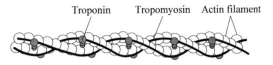

(C) Actin, troponin and tropomyosin

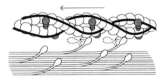

(D) Interaction of actin and myosin

Fig. 4.13. Myofibrillar molecules.

without moving your forearm. The globular head of myosin contains binding sites for interaction with the thin actin filaments of the sarcomere. The myosin head also contains an ATP-binding site that binds and hydrolyses ATP by its ATPase enzymatic activity. Myosin head ATPase is activated by ATP binding and degrades ATP to ADP, providing energy for the myosin heads to flex and move along the actin filaments during muscle contraction cycle. The golf club-shaped myosin molecules aggregate to form bundles of tail-to-tail polymers of many myosin molecules that form a feathered appearance, with the myosin heads projecting from the sides of the aggregate. These bundles of myosin molecules form the thick filaments of skeletal muscle.

Actin, the second most abundant protein in muscle cells, forms the thin filament of the sarcomere. The actin molecule consists of two strands of protein twisted upon one another, to form a rope-like, α-helical structure (Fig. 4.13). The long actin macromolecule is formed by a chain of multiple globular actin monomers, each of about 40 kDa in size. Actin contains the binding site for the myosin head. Two tropomyosin molecules twist around the length of the exterior of the actin molecule, residing in the groove formed between the two actin polymers. When the muscle is at rest, tropomyosin covers the myosin-binding site on actin. Another sarcomeric protein, troponin, binds to discrete sites on the tropomyosin molecule that occur at every seven actin monomers. Troponin consists of three subunits. One binds calcium during contraction (Tn-C), another is responsible for attaching troponin to tropomyosin (Tn-T) and the third, Tn-I, inhibits the interaction of actin and myosin. When calcium binds to the Tn-C subunit of troponin, troponin undergoes a conformational change. As a result, troponin pulls tropomyosin away from the actin–myosin-binding site on the actin molecule, exposing the myosin-binding sites on the actin molecule. Myosin can now bind to this site, flex and initiate muscle contraction. By pulling the actin molecules, immobilized at the Z-lines, toward the centre of the sarcomere, the sarcomeres are shortened, resulting in muscle contraction.

Another minor sarcomeric protein is titin, an elastic filament that connects the actin molecules to the borders of the sarcomere, the Z-discs. Titin is the largest known protein, composed of a long single chain of more than 27,000 amino acids that stretch for 1.5 μm. The titin molecule has a molecular weight of about 3 million Da. Titin is important in maintaining the passive tension of muscles at rest, may act as a molecular template for sarcomere organization and assists in the maintenance of the characteristic, highly organized structure of the sarcomere.

Myofibres and muscle contraction

Mature muscle fibres, or myofibres, are characterized by the presence of high proportions of mitochondria, which provide the energy, via oxidative phosphorylation of glucose, that is needed for muscle contraction. Mitochondria may account for more than 20% of the muscle cell volume in highly oxidative muscles. Much of the remainder of the muscle fibre consists of the insoluble protein molecules that are responsible for muscle contraction. Muscle cells secrete very little protein and this is reflected at the myofibre level by the low amount of endoplasmic reticulum within the cell. Most proteins are synthesized by ribosomes within the cytoplasm of the myofibre. The cytoplasm of the myofibre also contains energy reserves used for ATP generation that powers muscle contraction and cell metabolism. There are abundant glycogen granules near the sarcoplasmic reticulum and between myofibrils of the muscle cells. Lipid vacuoles are also present in cells that rely on oxidative metabolism.

Contraction of skeletal muscle is regulated by nerve impulses from motor neurones that form contacts, or synapses, with the muscle cells. Each muscle fibre is innervated by a motor neurone and the muscle fibre contracts in response to the release of the neurotransmitter, acetylcholine, by the motor neurones. A motor unit consists of a motor neurone and the muscle fibres that it innervates. In general, a single neurone will innervate about 150 muscle fibres. The plasma membrane of the myofibre is called the sarcolemma and invaginations of the sarcolemma form the transverse, or T-tubule structure that penetrates deep into the muscle fibre (Fig. 4.14). The T-tubule extension

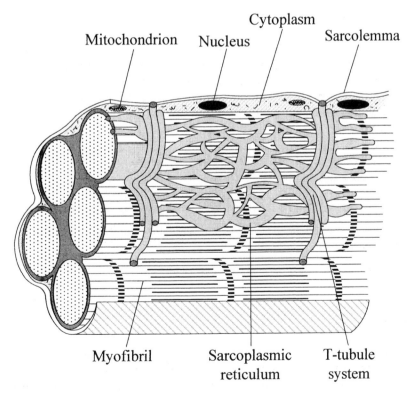

Fig. 4.14. Cross-section through a mature muscle cell.

of the sarcolemma provides a conduit for the neural activation signal into the cell's interior. This results in a more rapid response to stimulation than would be permitted by simple diffusion of molecules from the cell surface. Another specialized membrane within the muscle fibre, the sarcoplasmic reticulum, acts as a connection between the T-tubules and the contractile myofilaments. Calcium stored in the sarcoplasmic reticulum is released in response to nerve impulses from the T-tubules and is required for muscle contraction. The sarcoplasmic reticulum removes calcium from the myofilaments during muscle relaxation. Within the muscle, contraction is mediated by the myofibrils, which contain the contractile apparatus of the myofibre.

Muscle contraction is initiated by the release of acetylcholine into the neuromuscular junction. This results in the depolarization of the sarcolemma and this depolarization spreads to the interior of the myofibre via the intracellular T-tubule system. The membrane depolarization induces movement of calcium (Ca^{2+}) from the sarcoplasmic reticulum into the cytoplasm (Table 4.1). Calcium binds to the troponin C subunit, stimulating a conformational change in troponin. This results in the movement of tropomyosin away from myosin-binding sites on the actin molecule resulting in the exposure of the actin–myosin-binding sites on actin, allowing the formation of actin–myosin cross-bridges. The activated ATPase enzyme on the myosin head converts ATP to ADP and phosphate. The enzymatic conversion of ATP to ADP increases the affinity of myosin for actin and the energy produced is used to power the rapid conformational change in myosin around its hinge points, resulting in sliding of the attached thin actin filament towards the centre of the sarcomere. This results in a shortening of the sarcomere and muscle contraction. At the end of a contraction cycle, calcium is actively transported back into the sarcoplasmic reticulum, where it is no longer available to troponin. Tropomyosin then shields the actin–myosin-binding sites and the ATPase in the myosin head becomes inactive.

Table 4.1. The contraction cycle of skeletal muscle.

1. Cytosolic Ca^{2+} is increased

2. Troponin C binds Ca^{2+}, uncovers tropomyosin-shielded myosin-binding sites on actin

3. ATP bound to myosin head reduces the strength of actin–myosin binding, and the actin–myosin cross-bridge is broken

4. The unbound myosin head moves to a new actin-binding site and ATP is hydrolysed to ADP

5. The myosin head, with attached ADP, binds to a new actin site with high affinity

6. The actin–myosin cross-bridge generates

7. Myosin undergoes a rapid conformational change around its hinge points and ADP is released

8. The thin actin filament is pulled toward the M-line of the sarcomere

A single flexion of all actin–myosin contacts results in a muscle shortening of about 1%. As muscle contraction generally shortens muscles to about 30% of their resting length, the overall contraction is due to multiple attachment–release cycles between the actin and myosin molecules. The serial arrangement of the sarcomeres also contributes to the overall shortening, as the formation of the long myofilament composed of multiple repeating sarcomeric units allows the myofilament to act as a single unit, with the summation of single sarcomere shortenings, resulting in a longer overall shortening of the muscle. The contraction cycle continues as long as ATP and calcium are present. In the absence of ATP, the myosin head has a very high affinity for actin and is not released. This is the cause of post-mortem muscle shortening and the rigor mortis of muscle, which occurs after death.

Skeletal Muscle Fibre Types

Not all muscle fibres are equivalent. We are all familiar with the distinct dark and white meat of domestic poultry. The most basic classification of muscle fibres is based on this gross observation and was formalized in the 19th century. Dark meat has a higher proportion of red, slow twitch muscles, capable of sustained contraction. They are darker red than white muscle because of their abundance of myoglobin, an oxygen-carrying protein in muscle, and their highly vascularized nature. Red muscle fibres are involved in sustained, long-term activities such as standing and maintenance of posture. They are common in leg and back muscles. Although generally classified as slow twitch muscles, many red muscle fibres are fast twitch muscles. Large muscles that depend upon glycolysis for their energy have muscle fibre diameters that are generally larger than oxidative-type fibres. White muscle fibres, on the other hand, are considered fast twitch muscles, capable of quick reactions and using oxidative processes for energy production. Fast twitch muscles are used for sprinting, fine motor control and quick reflexive actions, have lower turnover rates and are more energy efficient. The gross classification of muscles into red or white types offers a simplified version of the muscle types. In reality, muscles contain a genetically determined, variable proportion of fast and slow twitch fibres. There is an almost continuous gradation of morphological, contractile and metabolic properties associated with muscles, but physiological and biochemical analysis of muscles allows us to classify muscle types into very few categories.

Physiological analyses of muscles provide ways to classify muscle fibres according to their functional characteristics. The contraction velocity, maximum contraction force and sustainability of that force, or fatigue resistance can be measured in experimental settings. These properties allow the characterization of the functional differences between muscles, but are difficult to obtain and require specialized equipment and training. These contractile characteristics are also reflected at the cellular and biochemical level, where differences in contraction velocities and relative oxidative vs glycolytic enzyme activities can be revealed by measuring the relative activities of enzymes involved in these processes. Characterization of muscle fibre types on the basis of their oxidative potential is done by the use of histochemical techniques. Staining of thin frozen sections of muscle with enzyme-specific reagents can be correlated with the physiological characteristics of a particular muscle. The use of these stains can reveal the proportion of fast and slow twitch fibres and the amount of oxidative vs non-oxidative muscle fibres in a particular muscle. Three muscle enzymes are used as markers to distinguish the characteristics of muscle fibres: myofibrillar ATPase, succinate dehydrogenase (SDH) and α-glycerophosphate dehydrogenase (αGPDH). Myofibrillar, or myosin, ATPase activity is proportional to the contraction velocity of a specific fibre and is used to distinguish between fast and slow twitch fibres. SDH is a mitochondrial enzyme that catalyses the conversion of succinate into fumarate during the Krebs, or citric acid cycle. Its presence is elevated in mitochondrial-rich cells and indicates a high level of oxidative metabolism. The last enzyme used in fibre typing, αGPDH, is located in the cytoplasm and is a measure of the glycolytic, or anaerobic, metabolism of the cell. The use of these histochemical stains can be used to classify muscle fibres into fast or slow, oxidative or non-oxidative, and glycolytic or non-glycolytic. Using these three stains provides eight (2^3) different possible fibre types, but more than 95% of muscle fibres can be categorized into only three major groups. These three muscle types are: (i) fast glycolytic (FG) fibres with high levels of αGPDH and ATPase; (ii) fast oxidative-glycolytic (FOG) fibres containing high levels of all three markers; and (iii) slow oxidative (SO) fibres having high levels of SDH, but low levels of ATPase and αGPDH (Table 4.2).

A more recent muscle typing method uses immunohistochemical (IHC) methods to distinguish between different isoforms of the MHC. Using monoclonal antibodies directed toward specific sites on the MHC and comparing results with fibres stained for the histochemical markers, four different fibre types could be distinguished, one correlating with the slow twitch fibre type and three with the fast twitch fibre types. Type 1 MHC fibres are found in slow twitch muscles and cardiac muscle, type 2A MHC is in most FOG muscles. Types 2B and 2X are typical of FG muscle fibres and are fairly rare, found only in extraocular, laryngeal and jaw muscles. Fibre type 2X is classified as a muscle fibre type that displays properties intermediate between those of 2A and 2B. The 2X fibre types represent a small population of skeletal muscle fibres that do not readily fit into the other categories (Table 4.2).

Table 4.2. Skeletal muscle fibre types.

Twitch/metabolism	MHC type	ATPase	SDH	GPDH
Slow oxidative (SO)	Type 1	+	++++	+
Fast oxidative-glycolytic (FOG)	Type 2A	++++	++++	++++
Fast glycolytic (FG)	Type 2B	++++	+	++++
Fast intermediate (FG)	Type 2X	++++	+	++++

Skeletal muscle protein turnover

While the number and size of skeletal muscle cells are important factors in the determination of skeletal muscle growth and ultimate size, the rates of skeletal muscle protein turnover are also essential for muscle growth. Skeletal muscle protein levels result from a balance between protein synthesis and protein degradation. Different rates of skeletal muscle growth are dependent upon regulation of muscle cell protein degradation to a greater extent than the rates of protein synthesis. Protein accumulation in muscle cells occurs in an environment in which degradation is inhibited and synthesized proteins can accumulate in the cell. In addition, the contractile myofibrillar proteins have a finite lifespan and, like any cellular component, must be degraded and replaced by newly synthesized proteins. Intracellular enzymes called calpains play a prominent role in maintaining the balance between muscle protein degradation and synthesis.

Calpains are calcium-dependent proteolytic enzymes found in all vertebrate cells studied and are especially important in the regulation of skeletal muscle protein degradation. Two forms of these enzymes are present in muscle cells, distinguished by the concentrations of calcium required to activate them. The m-calpains require 400 to 800 µM Ca^{2+} for activation, while the µ-calpains are activated by lower levels of calcium, 3 to 5 µM. Binding to other proteins called calpastatins inactivates the calpains. Calpains degrade specific muscle proteins, such as titin, desmin and troponin T as well as other minor skeletal muscle proteins. Myosin is degraded slowly and incompletely by calpains and actin is unaffected by these proteases. The effects of calpains on the degradation of minor proteins of the sarcomere results in the loss of Z-discs from the sarcomere. This is due in part to the cleavage of the N-terminal (Z-disc) end of the titin molecule that connects actin to the Z-line. Calpains do not completely degrade proteins into small polypeptides and amino acids. Calpain degradation results in the generation of large polypeptide chains that are then degraded to amino acids by lysosomal proteases, the cathepsins. Calpains also degrade certain cytoplasmic enzymes such as most protein kinases and phosphatases, leading to speculation that calpains may have indirect regulatory functions within the cell, as kinases and phosphatases activate and inactivate a variety of intracellular proteins.

While concentrations of calpains within the cell remain relatively constant, calpastatin levels fluctuate with physiological states. For example, in animals treated with β-agonists, muscle protein hypertrophy is stimulated while levels of calpastatin increase several fold. This is believed to inhibit calpain proteolysis and allow the accumulation of muscle protein. Likewise, calpastatin activity is increased in specific muscles that undergo hypertrophy as a result of the Callipyge gene in sheep. These animals have a 30% to 50% increase in the muscle mass of skeletal muscles in the hind limb and back regions. Calpastatin activity is increased specifically in these muscles, but not in muscles that are unaffected by the Callipyge gene. Again, the accumulation of protein in hypertrophied muscles is believed to result from reduced protein degradation in the muscle cell as calpain activity is reduced by elevated calpastatin activity. Calpains are important in the post-mortem tenderization of meat. Ninety-five per cent of the muscle protein proteolysis that occurs in the first 1 to 2 weeks after slaughter is due to activation of skeletal muscle calpains upon death of the animal.

The formation of multinucleated skeletal muscle cells

In biology, we now know many things that we take for granted. For example, we have known for many years that skeletal muscle cells were multi-nucleated. However, the mechanism by which these cells became multinucleated was not known. Were the nuclei the result of replication of nuclei within a single cell without cell division, a process called endoredu-plication, or did the multiple nuclei result from fusion of many mononucle-ated precursor cells? In the mid-1960s, Beatrice Mintz set out to answer this question using a sophisticated approach.

This study used mice from two different strains, one with a black fur coat and one white. These strains carry different forms (isozymes) of the enzyme isocitrate dehydrogenase (IDH). IDH consists of two protein chains that are unique to the particular isozyme. The chemical differences in the IDH isozymes result in different mobilities in an electric field, and the isozymes could be distinguished from each other after separation by elec-trophoresis. Critical to the design of this study is the ability of these protein chains to combine with one another in the cytoplasm to form hybrids of the isozyme. These hybrid IDH molecules consist of a protein chain from each of the isozymes. When subjected to electrophoresis, hybrid molecules migrate a distance that is intermediate to that of the original IDH isozymes. Thus, if the isozymes were from several genetically different nuclei, as expected in the fusion model, an intermediate hybrid form (a/b) of the enzyme would be present (Fig. 4.15). If the multinucleated cells were derived from a single nucleus by endoreduplication, cells would contain only one type of IDH gene and only the original forms (a/a or b/b) of the isozymes would be present.

Drs Mintz and Baker created a new, mosaic animal by combining the blastomeres of early, undifferentiated embryos from each of the strains. These chimeric embryos, which the authors called tetraparental or allophenic mice, were then transferred into recipient dams and allowed to come to full term. Successful allophenic mice were phenotypically distin-guished from the original black or white strains by their patched black and white coat colour. Skeletal muscle and liver (used as a control, mononucle-ated tissue) were collected for electrophoretic analysis of isozyme patterns. Isozyme patterns were compared with conventional reproductive crosses between the strains of mice. As shown in Fig. 4.16, skeletal muscle from con-ventional matings and from the allophenic mice contained the original isozymes as well as the intermediate form. This combination of all three combinations of IDH isozymes was expected if multinucleation resulted from fusion of myoblasts containing different IDH alleles. The IDH isozyme

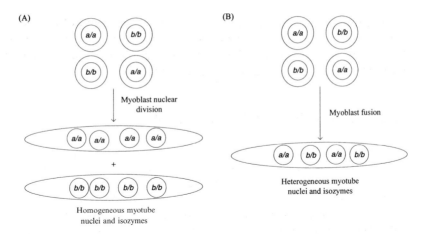

Fig. 4.15. Two models that may account for the formation of multinucleated myotubes.

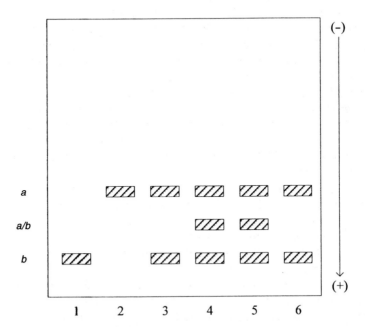

Fig. 4.16. Pattern of IDH enzyme activity observed after electrophoretic separation of tissues isolated from skeletal muscle (SM) or liver (L): 1, IDH strain *b*, SM or L; 2, IDH strain *a*, SM or L; 3, pooled tissue of strain *a* and strain *b*, SM or L; 4, F$_1$ cross of IDH strain *a* plus IDH strain *b*, SM or L; 5, allophenic (chimeric) strain *a/b* SM; 5, allophenic strain *a/b*, L. The arrow on the right indicates the direction of electrophoresis. Source: Mintz and Baker (1967).

pattern of mononucleated liver tissue from allophenic mice, however, displayed only the original isozyme patterns. This was the expected result from a tissue that contained the isozyme alleles in separate cells. Liver tissue from conventional matings, in which genes from both parents are present in a single nucleus, also contained the intermediate hybrid form of the IDH enzyme. Thus, it was established that multinucleated skeletal muscle cells were derived from fusion of many precursor cells and not from the replication of a single nucleus within a precursor cell.

Adipose Tissue Growth and Development

We are all familiar with adipose tissue, or fat, both on a personal level and on a nutritional level. Diet-induced obesity and the accompanying Type II diabetes are common in the human populations of Western Europe and the USA and are prominent health concerns in these countries. Likewise, when we consume meat products, we savour the flavours imparted by the adipose tissue, which is part of all meats. In animal production, fat is an important component of edible meat, but is an expensive addition. The deposition of appropriate quantities of fat in an animal destined for consumption is an important component of the costs of animal production and the suitability of the product for human consumption. The length of time taken to fatten food animals is a major cost for producers. On the other hand, the accumulation of intramuscular fat increases the quality and value of the meat product.

Fat is an energy-dense tissue. When consumed, the lipids in fat produce roughly 9 kcal/g, while those of protein and carbohydrate produce about 4 kcal/g. This means, of course, that the biological synthesis of lipids also requires over twice the amount of food energy than carbohydrate or protein. Thus, the deposition of fat is a costly enterprise, both metabolically and economically. A great deal of the subcutaneous fat deposited in food animals is wasted, as it is trimmed from carcasses and discarded or used as the basis to make products of lesser value. It has been estimated that the USA produces over 2 billion kilograms of excess lipid each year from the production of food animals. Because of the economic importance of adipose tissue and the negative economic impact of excess subcutaneous adipose tissue deposition, knowledge of the developmental and cellular processes of fat formation is essential to understand the regulation of fat deposition and to eventually improve farm animal production efficiency.

Brown adipose tissue

Mammalian adipose tissue exists in two forms, white adipose tissue, the most common form, and brown adipose tissue. Brown adipose tissue is found in various locations, which are species-dependent. While the primary role of white adipose tissue is energy storage, brown adipose tissue is adapted for energy use and heat production. Brown adipose tissue is richly vascularized and contains abundant mitochondria for energy production from lipid and glucose catabolism. Brown adipose tissue is also characterized by the presence of high levels of the protein, uncoupling protein-1 (UCP1), which functions to uncouple mitochondrial oxidative phosphorylation from ATP production. This results in the release of energy in the form of heat. This is known as non-shivering thermogenesis and brown adipose tissue is the sole source. Heat produced by non-shivering thermogenesis is essential to maintain homeostatic body temperature in neonatal animals and in animals emerging from hibernation. This ensures neonatal survival and survival in cold climates. At birth, with the exception of subcutaneous fat, essentially all adipose tissue in cattle and sheep can be considered to be brown adipose tissue. Brown adipose tissue in newborn sheep and cattle is replaced by white adipose tissue within the first week of neonatal life. This occurs without a change in adipocyte cell numbers and is believed to result from transdifferentiation of brown adipocytes into white adipocytes. In the adult, brown adipose tissue responds to environmental and nutritional cues. For example, in adult rats, brown adipose tissue depots undergo enlargement via hyperplasia in response to cold acclimation and to increased food intake. Activation of brown adipose tissue thermogenesis is controlled by norepinephrine release from the sympathetic nervous system (SNS).

White adipose tissue

White adipose tissue is the tissue we generally think of as fat and is the subject of this section. White adipose tissue is the major storage site for energy in the form of lipid, when dietary energy sources exceed energy use by the animal. This energy reserve can be used during times of food scarcity. In addition, subcutaneous white adipose tissue provides a layer of insulation that prevents heat loss in cold environments. Many internal organs are surrounded by a layer of visceral fat that provides a mechanical cushion to protect organs against physical trauma. Since the discovery in 1994 that white adipose tissue secretes the hormone leptin, adipose tissue has been recognized as an endocrine tissue. Adipose tissue is no longer considered as just a relatively passive storage reservoir, but is involved in regulation of appetite, reproduction and energy homeostasis. The endocrine function of adipose tissue will be discussed in subsequent chapters.

Fat is a diffuse organ that is present in several discrete sites, or depots, throughout the body. Fat depots are present in many visceral sites in association with the internal organs. For example, fat is found as perirenal, omental, cardiac and mesenteric depots. Fat also develops in association with internal reproductive organs such as the uterus (parametrial) and the testes (epididymal). Subcutaneous fat, located between the muscle and skin of animals, is the most easily identified and morphologically visible of the fat depots. In addition, fat infiltrates muscles, where it is found as intermuscular or seam fat, between large muscle groups and within muscles as intramuscular fat. Developmentally, the visceral fat depots are formed first, followed by the subcutaneous fat depot, and finally, in adulthood, intra-muscular fat is formed. Depot sites are constant in mammals, but proportions vary with species. For example, subcutaneous fat is much more prominent in pigs than in beef cattle and relatively sparse in dairy cattle. Likewise, beef cattle have much more abdominal fat than dairy cattle.

White adipose tissue consists primarily of lipid (76–94%) and, like bone, is classified as a connective tissue. Nearly 90% to 99% of lipid in the adipocyte consists of triacylglycerols, with small amounts of free fatty acids, phospholipids, mono- and diacylglycerols and cholesterol. Adipose tissue is composed of two distinct components: the lipid-containing fat cells or adipocytes and the non-lipid component, the stromovascular cells. The stromovascular portion of adipose tissue consists of a variety of blood cells, fibroblasts, endothelial cells, pericytes and adipocyte precursor cells. The stromovascular cell fraction of adipose tissue provides an important reservoir of stem cells for production of new adipocytes. Adipocyte precursor cells can be isolated from the stromovascular cell fraction of the neonatal, adult and even senescent animal. These preadipocytes can be grown *in vitro* and are important sources of cells to study the regulation of adipocyte differentiation.

Adipose tissue development

Adipocytes develop from embryonic mesenchymal cells beginning in mid to late gestation in mammals. The specific time of initiation of adipocyte formation varies with the depot site and the species studied. In the fetus, adipogenesis occurs in close association with vascular development. In the adult, fat is highly vascularized and each adult adipocyte is in contact with at least one capillary. Adipocyte precursor cells aggregate as fat cell clusters in fat depot sites that surround existing capillary beds. These fat primordia increase in size and number during fetal development and undergo rapid expansion in the neonatal animal. The increase in neonatal adipose mass is the result of hyperplasia of precursor cells combined with hypertrophy of existing adipocytes. Most of the body's fat reserves develop postnatally. At birth, the bodies of farm animals contain roughly 1–4% fat, while at maturity, these animals can have as much as 40% of their body weight as fat.

In the adult, adipocyte precursor cells are derived either from the circulation, adjacent tissues or the stromovascular cells of the adipose tissue. It is not clear if the stem cell is a fibroblast, macrophage or blood vessel pericyte. In any case, stem cell replication produces adipoblasts, which are morphologically indistinguishable from other cells, but are committed to the adipocyte lineage. Adipoblasts replicate and differentiate into preadipocytes (Fig. 4.17). Again, newly formed preadipocytes are not morphologically distinct from other cells, but as preadipocytes differentiate, they are characterized by the accumulation of small lipid droplets and the appearance of lipogenic enzymes. An early marker of differentiation is lipoprotein lipase (LPL), whose function is to assist in the accumulation of lipids in the cell.

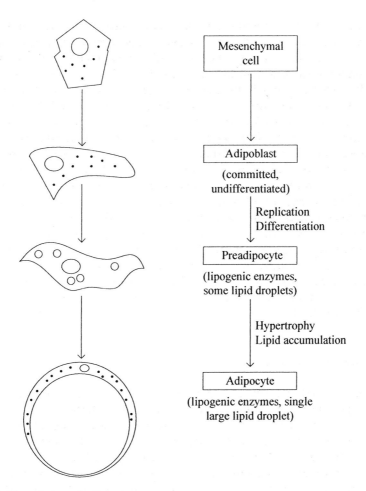

Fig. 4.17. Differentiation of adipocytes.

After lipid filling and cellular enlargement the cell assumes the typical 'signet ring' morphology of the mature adipocyte. This results from the accumulation of a large lipid droplet within the cell that forces the cytoplasm and nucleus of the adipocyte to the periphery. The cell is now capable of expression of the full complement of enzymes that catalyse lipogenesis, such as fatty acid synthase (FAS), pyruvate carboxylase and acetyl-CoA carboxylase (ACC).

Adipose tissue growth: hyperplasia vs hypertrophy

How do adult animals accumulate large amounts of fat? Up until the mid-1970s, it was thought that a specific number of fat cells was present at birth and the number of adipocytes did not change during the lifetime of the animal. This was supported by the observation that mature adipocytes were incapable of mitosis. It is now known that fat accretion in the adult is a function not only of lipid accumulation and an increase in adipocyte size, or hypertrophy, but also as a result of an increase in fat cell numbers by hyperplasia.

In the adolescent animal, nutrition and exercise affect adipocyte numbers. These changes in adipocyte cell numbers persist into adulthood. In the adult, early observations suggested that total cell number in adipose tissue depots were constant and unaffected by typical regulators of cell growth such as nutrition, exercise and hormones. These observations gave rise to an early theory of adipose tissue accumulation called the *critical period theory* that divided the growth of adipose tissue into two phases. The first is the developmentally early, sensitive, pre-adult phase, characterized by marked adipoblast hyperplasia and sensitivity to external stimuli. This is followed by the adult phase, characterized by stable, unchanging adipocyte cell numbers. In the adult phase, adipocyte growth was thought to occur solely by the accumulation of lipids, or fat cell hypertrophy, the enlargement of fat cells. This early work was criticized on several points, many of them apparent in hindsight, after the development of more sophisticated methods to study adipocytes. For example, early studies used inadequate methods to count adipose cells; rats and hamsters, which are now known to be unique in their absence of adult cell division, were used as model organisms; and depots, which are not representative of overall fat growth, were studied. For example, most of the early studies used rodent epididymal fat as an epididymal fat depot model. While this depot is abundant and readily accessible in rodents, epididymal fat is not representative of adipose tissue growth seen in subcutaneous and visceral fat.

It is now known that the number of adipocytes is not fixed at birth and that adult adipose depots increase in size by mechanisms which involve both hyperplasia and hypertrophy. Faust and co-workers postulated the *maximum fat cell size theory* in 1978. This theory posits that adipocyte numbers initially stabilize at a certain level before maturity. During this phase, cell numbers are constant but adipose cells accumulate lipid and cell size continues to increase. When a certain 'maximum fat cell size' is reached in early adulthood, new fat cells are recruited from stem cells or adipoblast precursors (Fig. 4.18). Evidence now exists that when adipocytes reach a certain maximal size, they secrete growth factors and other paracrine agents that

Fig. 4.18. Changes in fat cell size and numbers during postnatal life. Adapted from Johnson and Francendese (1985).

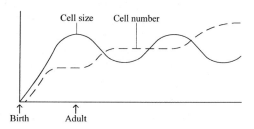

stimulate the growth and differentiation of adipocyte stem cells in the stromovascular fraction of adipose tissue. This will be discussed in a later chapter that deals with the regulation of adipocyte development. Recruitment of new cells results in an increase in fat cell numbers. Addition of these new undifferentiated cells to the fat depot reduces the average fat cell size in the adipose depot. This cycle of adipocyte hypertrophy and hyperplasia can be repeated several times during adulthood and senescence, with the volume of fat cells reaching a maximum again and again, followed by the recruitment of new fat cell precursors for addition to the adipocyte depot. This theory provides a more flexible, realistic picture of fat cell development in the adult and has generated new interest in the study of fat cell morphogenesis and its regulation.

Lipogenesis and Lipolysis

Adipose tissue plays an essential role in the storage and release of energy by sequestering and mobilizing fat, or triacylglycerols. The adipocyte is the primary cell that stores fats, and fats are constantly degraded and resynthesized in the adipocyte. The main storage form of fat is triacylglycerol, a macromolecule consisting of a glycerol backbone esterified to three long chains of fatty acids. Triacylglycerols may be supplied to adipocytes from the liver and the intestine in the form of serum lipoproteins. These complexes of fat and protein appear in the circulation as chylomicrons, from intestinal absorption, or as high, low or very low-density lipoproteins (abbreviated HDL, LDL and VLDL, respectively) derived from the liver.

LPL, an enzyme synthesized by many tissues and localized on the endothelial cell surface of capillaries, catalyses the removal of fatty acids from the lipoproteins. After the fatty acids enter the cell, they are reconverted to triacylglycerols by adipocytes. Triacylglycerols may also be synthesized from circulating free (i.e. non-esterified) fatty acids that circulate in the bloodstream bound to albumin. After their uptake by the cell they are esterified to glycerol to form triacylglycerols (Figs. 4.19 and 4.20). These mechanisms of triacylglycerol formation are common in many omnivores or carnivores that consume diets relatively high in lipids. In animals that consume small amounts of lipids (as well as omnivores and carnivores) long-chain fatty acids may also be synthesized *de novo* by the process called lipogenesis. Lipogenesis *per se* involves the synthesis of fatty acids from small, unrelated precursor molecules that are derived from rumenal fermentation or glycolysis of sugars. The conjugation of fatty acids to glycerol to form triacylglycerols is a process separate from lipogenesis.

In humans and birds, lipogenesis occurs primarily in the liver. In ruminants and pigs, the adipocyte is the main site for lipogenesis. Fatty acids are synthesized from the two-carbon precursors, acetate or lactate, or from glucose after it has been converted to pyruvate by glycolysis (Fig. 4.21). While glucose is the primary precursor of fatty acids in non-ruminants, microbial catabolism of glucose in the rumen of ruminants results in the production of

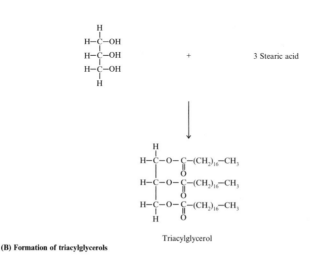

Oleic acid

Palmitic acid

(A) Examples of fatty acids

3 Stearic acid

Triacylglycerol

(B) Formation of triacylglycerols

Fig. 4.19. Fatty acids and the formation of triacylglycerols.

pyruvate and acetate. Acetate is the major precursor for lipogenesis in these animals. The synthesis of long-chain fatty acids occurs in the cytoplasm by the repeated addition of two carbons to a 'primer' molecule, which is usually acetyl-coenzyme A (acetyl-CoA).

ACC is the enzyme that catalyses the initial, rate-limiting step of lipogenesis. This results in the conversion of acetyl-CoA to malonyl-CoA. Malonyl-CoA then acts as the donor of two-carbon acetyl groups to the growing fatty acid chain. Increased circulating insulin concentrations, in response to dietary energy, induce ACC gene transcription and translation resulting in an increase in ACC and increased rates of lipogenesis and fatty acid formation. The insulin counter-regulatory hormones, glucagon, epinephrine and norepinephrine, inhibit the activity of ACC. This occurs in times of fat mobilization during times of food shortage or in stressful situations.

After the formation of malonyl-CoA, FAS catalyses the remainder of the lipogenic cycle. FAS is a large macromolecular complex (MW ~500,000) con-

Name	Number of carbons	
	Number of double bonds	
	Position of double bonds	
Formic acid	1: 0	
Acetic acid	2: 0	
Propionic acid	3: 0	
Butyric acid	4: 0	
Valerianic acid	5: 0	
Caproic acid	6: 0	
Caprylic acid	8: 0	
Capric acid	10: 0	
Lauric acid	12: 0	
Myristic acid	14: 0	
Palmitic acid	16: 0	
Stearic acid	18: 0	
Oleic acid	18: 1; 9	
Linoleic acid	18: 2; 9,12	
Linolenic acid	18: 3; 9,12,15	
Arachidic acid	20: 0	
Arachidonic acid	20: 4; 5,8,11,14	

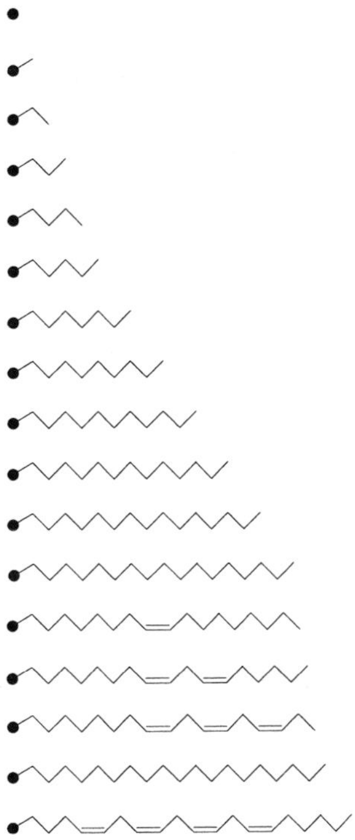

Fig. 4.20. Structure and nomenclature of fatty acids.

sisting of two identical protein subunits, arranged head-to-tail. Each subunit contains seven different catalytic activities and the molecular arrangement of the homodimers allows FAS to catalyse the simultaneous synthesis of two fatty acid chains. Although FAS is not a rate-limiting enzyme for lipogenesis, it is essential for the chain elongation of fatty acids. The overall equation for the synthesis of palmitic acid (a 16-carbon fatty acid) is:

$$\text{Acetyl-CoA} + 7\text{malonyl-CoA} + 14\text{NADPH} + 14\text{H}^+$$
$$\rightarrow \text{Palmitic acid} + 7\text{CO}_2 + 8\text{CoA} + 14\text{NADP}^+ + 6\text{H}_2\text{O}$$

Palmitic acid is the primary product of lipogenesis in adipose tissue. It is converted to the 18-carbon stearic acid (C-18) in the endoplasmic reticulum by the enzyme fatty acid elongase. Stearoyl-CoA desaturase (SCD or Δ9 desaturase) converts a portion of stearic acid into oleic acid, the 18-carbon non-saturated form of stearic acid, by the insertion of a double bond between carbons 9 and 10. The presence of oleic acid, which has a lower melting point than stearic acid, ensures the fluidity of lipids.

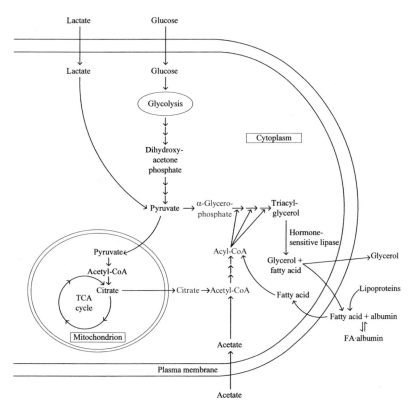

Fig. 4.21. Lipid metabolism.

The long-chain fatty acids that are synthesized during lipogenesis are then esterified to a glycerol backbone. Concentrations of non-esterified fatty acids are very low in the body and the formation of triacylglycerols provides a non-toxic storage form for lipids. In ruminants, non-saturated fats derived from the diet are quickly hydrogenated to saturated fats in the rumen before intestinal absorption and, as a result, ruminant fatty acids are, in general, more saturated than those of non-ruminants.

Mobilization of fat stores occurs when dietary energy intake is reduced or when the animal is subjected to stress. An overall view of lipid metabolism is given in Fig. 4.21. The process of lipolysis is initiated by the sequential release of fatty acids from the glycerol backbone of triglycerols. The initial lipolytic event is catalysed by hormone-sensitive lipase, an enzyme that is activated by the hormone messenger, cAMP. The primary hormonal inducers of lipolysis in mammals are the catecholamines, epinephrine and norepinephrine. In birds, glucagon is the main inducer of hormone-sensitive lipase. The activity of hormone-sensitive lipase determines the amount of fatty acids released by adipocytes. Thus, this enzyme is the major determinant of blood lipid levels. Long-chain fatty acids released from adipose tis-

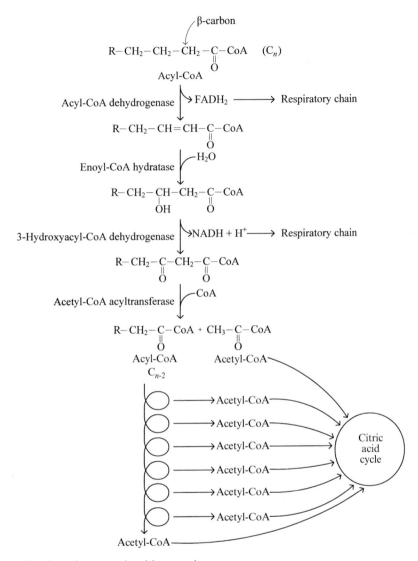

Fig. 4.22. The β-oxidation cycle of fatty acids.

sue into the systemic circulation are only slightly soluble in water. Therefore, they circulate bound to albumin in the bloodstream.

Fatty acids from the circulation are taken up by cells to resynthesize fats or to generate energy by fatty acid catabolism. Degradation of fatty acids occurs in the mitochondria by a process known as β-oxidation. Cleavage of the long-chain fatty acids occurs at the carboxyl end of the fatty acid between carbon-2 (the α-carbon) and carbon-3 (the β-carbon), hence the name β-oxidation (Fig. 4.22). This occurs after binding of fatty acids to coenzyme A in the cytoplasm. The activated fatty acid (acyl-CoA) is then transported into the mitochondria via the carnitine shuttle system. In the mitochondria, the long-chain fatty acids are sequentially degraded to two-carbon acetyl-CoA residues. The complete oxidation of a long-chain fatty acid requires several trips through the β-oxidation cycle. For example, eight cycles are required for the oxidation of stearic acid, an 18-carbon fatty acid. The acetate molecules, in the form of acetyl-CoA, then enter the citric acid cycle and the respiratory chain to undergo final oxidation to CO_2 with a concomitant production of ATP. The energy balance for the complete oxidation of palmitic acid (16:0) is shown in Fig. 4.23. A total of 106 ATP are produced per molecule of palmitic acid, for a free energy gain of 3300 kJ/mol. The amount of energy from the degradation of fatty acids is much greater than from the degradation of carbohydrates (32 ATP per molecule of glucose) or from proteins, even when the different sizes of the molecules is considered. This demonstrates the superiority of the use of fat as an energy storage molecule.

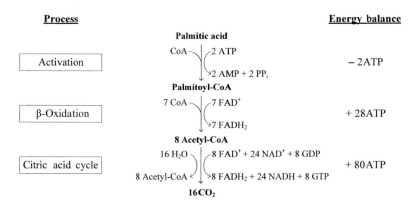

Fig. 4.23. Summary of the energy produced from fatty acid degradation.

References and Further Reading

Ailhaud, G., Grimaldi, P. and Negrel, R. (1992) Cellular and molecular aspects of adipose tissue development. *Annual Review of Nutrition* 12, 207–233.

Allen, R.E., Merkel, R.A. and Young, R.B. (1979) Cellular aspects of muscle growth: myogenic cell proliferation. *Journal of Animal Science* 49, 115–127.

Brook, C.G.D. (1972) Evidence for a sensitive period in adipose cell replication in man. *Lancet* ii, 624.

Drackley, J.K. (2000) Lipid metabolism. In: D'Mello, J.P.F. (ed.) *Farm Animal Metabolism and Nutrition.* CAB International, Wallingford, UK, pp. 97–119.

Faust, I.M., Johnson, P.R., Stern, J.J. and Hirsch, J. (1978) Diet-induced adipocyte number increase in adult rats: a new model of obesity. *American Journal of Physiology* 235, E279.

Goll, D.E., Thompson, V.F., Taylor, R.G. and Ouali, A. (1998) The calpain system and skeletal muscle growth. *Canadian Journal of Animal Science* 78, 503–512.

Johnson, P.R. and Francendese, A.A. (1985) Cellular regulation of adipose tissue growth. *Journal of Animal Science* 61(Suppl. 2), 57–75.

Lieber, R.L. (2002) *Skeletal Muscle Structure, Function and Plasticity.* Lippincott, Williams & Wilkins, Philadelphia, Pennsylvania, 369 pp.

Mersmann, H.J. (1991) Regulation of adipose tissue metabolism and accretion in mammals raised for meat production. In: Pearson, A.M. and Dutson, T.R. (eds) *Advances in Meat Research*, Vol. 7. Elsevier Applied Science, New York, pp. 135–168.

Mintz, B. and Baker, W.B. (1967) Normal mammalian muscle differentiation and gene control of isocitrate dehydrogenase synthesis. *Proceedings of the National Academy of Sciences USA* 58, 592–598.

Nakagawa, N., Kinosaki, M., Yamaguchi, K., Shima, N., Yasuda, H., Yano, K., Morinaga, T. and Higashio, K. (1998) RANK is the essential signaling receptor for osteoclast differentiation factor in osteoclastogenesis. *Biochemical and Biophysical Research Communications* 253, 395–400.

Takahashi, N., Udagawa, N., Takami, M. and Suda, T. (2002) Cells of bone, osteoclast generation. In: Bilezikian, J.P., Raisz, L.G. and Rodan, G.A. (eds) *Principles of Bone Biology*, Vol. 1, 2nd edn. Academic Press, New York, pp. 109–126.

5 Growth Hormone and Insulin-like Growth Factors

Evans and Simpson first discovered a pituitary factor that enhances animal growth in the 1920s when a bovine pituitary extract was shown to promote growth in rats. Based on this observation, the activity was termed 'growth hormone' (GH). Later studies in the following decade demonstrated that the anterior pituitary extracts also had metabolic effects; reducing carcass fat and increasing milk yield in treated animals. Isolation of GH from anterior pituitary glands was accomplished in 1945 and its activity in promoting growth and lactation was correlated to the original crude anterior pituitary gland extracts.

Advances in molecular biology and genetic engineering in the late 1970s and early 1980s allowed the use of recombinant DNA to produce large amounts of bovine GH (bGH) from bacterial plasmids containing the bGH gene. The availability of large quantities of bGH provided enough bGH, and later porcine GH (pGH), to be used in studies of the effects of GH in large domestic animals. The availability of GH for studies in large farm animals has provided a wealth of information about the effects of GH on physiological processes in ruminant and non-ruminant animals. These basic studies, in turn, have led to the commercialization of the use of GH to promote lactation in dairy cattle.

It is now known that many of the effects of GH are indirect, as one of the major target organs of GH is the liver. Under GH stimulation, the liver synthesizes and secretes IGF-I, which acts as a hormone to induce many of the effects that were originally believed to be direct effects of GH on other target tissues such as muscle, bone and adipose tissue. The aim of this chapter is to first examine the biochemistry, mechanism of action and metabolic effects of GH and then to outline the IGF system and its physiological effects. Finally, studies on the effects of GH and IGF-I treatment of farm animals will be discussed.

The GH Molecule

GH, also called somatotropin (ST), is synthesized and secreted by the somatotrope cells of the anterior pituitary gland. It is a single-chain protein with a molecular weight of about 22,000. In most species, GH consists of 191 amino acids and contains two disulphide bonds that maintain its three-dimensional structure. The amino acid sequence of GH is similar to prolactin (PRL) and placental lactogen (PL) (Fig. 5.1). PRL is a hormone that is primarily involved in the induction of milk synthesis in mammals. PL is synthesized in the placenta during pregnancy and is thought to be a regulator of fetal glucose supply, maternal mammogenesis, and in some species, fetal growth. Due to this overlapping amino acid homology, PRL, PL and GH have overlapping biological actions.

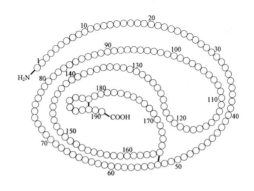

Growth hormone

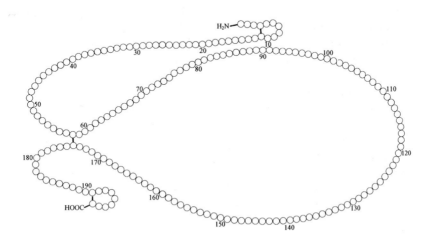

Prolactin

Fig. 5.1. Structures of growth hormone and prolactin. Both have two cysteines that form intramolecular covalent disulphide bonds, 190 to 200 amino acids and regions of identical amino acid sequences.

Control of GH secretion

Circulating concentrations of GH vary widely. The secretion of GH from the anterior pituitary is pulsatile, and GH concentrations in plasma occur as irregular spikes of concentration followed by very low levels of GH. The specific pattern of GH release is related to the species, sex and age of the animal. Spikes in GH concentrations occur roughly six to eight times during a 24 h period. For this reason, the accurate measurement of blood GH concentrations is difficult and time-consuming. Single blood samples, sufficient for quantitation of other hormones, are inadequate to measure GH and lead to samples with wide variations of GH concentrations. Sequential blood samples, taken at 15 or 20 min intervals over a 6 to 8 h period are required to establish a useful record of overall GH concentrations. When GH concentrations are measured, data are accumulated on overall, mean GH concentration, frequency of GH pulses and high and low GH levels. The actions of GH are believed to be dependent upon not only overall concentrations, but also maximum GH pulse levels and the frequency of GH secretory pulses. Enhanced effects on growth promotion are seen when GH is administered in multiple, small doses rather than as a large, single, daily injection or a continuous infusion. This is an impractical treatment in animal production systems, but reflects the endogenous rhythms and complex mechanisms that regulate animal growth in the intact system.

The release of GH from the anterior pituitary gland is influenced by several physiological factors, including neurotransmitters, hypothalamic peptides and circulating metabolites. Specific CNS neurotransmitters that affect the hypothalamus such as serotonin precursors, GABA and dopamine alter GH release. Reduced levels of blood glucose (hypoglycaemia) and concomitant elevations of blood insulin induce GH release. High concentrations of circulating amino acids, especially arginine, induce GH release, while elevated levels of circulating IGF-I, free fatty acids and obesity inhibit GH secretion. GH levels are increased during the physiological states of sleep, stress, exercise and starvation.

As with all anterior pituitary hormones, the secretion of GH is controlled by the hypothalamus (Fig. 5.2). The hypothalamus produces peptides that stimulate and inhibit the release of GH from the anterior pituitary. Traditionally, two hypothalamic peptides, one stimulating and one inhibiting GH release, were believed to be the only controls of GH release. It is now known that additional hypothalamic peptides are involved in the control of GH release from the anterior pituitary.

The release of GH from the anterior pituitary is induced by hypothalamic GHRH. GHRH is a 44-amino acid peptide synthesized by cells in the arcuate (ARC) nucleus of the hypothalamus (Fig. 5.3). GHRH is secreted from neurosecretory nerve terminals in the median eminence and transported to the anterior pituitary gland by the hypophyseal portal system. GHRH binds to a G-linked protein receptor in somatotropes, stimulating an increase in cAMP and activating GH release via the transcription factor, pit-1.

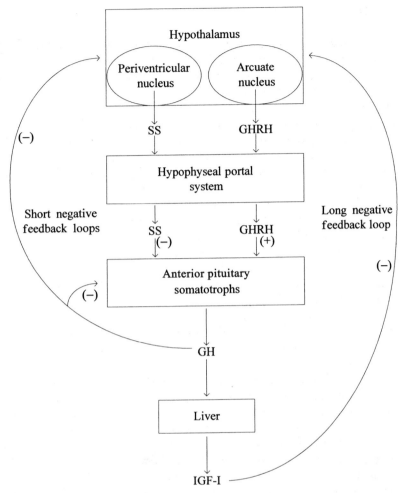

Fig. 5.2. Hypothalamic control and negative feedback loops for the regulation of GH secretion.

Somatostatin (SS) or GHRIH is produced in the periventricular nucleus of the hypothalamus. It is a tetradecapeptide (14 amino acids) that is found in many tissues outside the hypothalamus. This includes the CNS and delta cells of endocrine pancreas and gut. As the name implies, SS inhibits the release of GH from the anterior pituitary by reducing cAMP concentrations within the somatotropes. In addition, it inhibits TRH-induced release of TSH (but not TRH-induction of PRL release). SS also acts as an inhibitor of several other hormones and metabolites including PTH, calcitonin, gastric HCl, acetylcholine and catecholamine neurotransmitters.

Although TRH is the primary hypothalamic peptide that induces pituitary TSH release, it also induces GH release in birds, cattle and rats. TRH is a tripeptide [(pyro)glu-his-pro-amide] produced in the paraventricular

Tyr–Ala–Asp–Ala–Ile–Phe –Thr–Asn–Ser –Tyr–Arg–Lys–Val–Leu–Gly–Gln–Leu–Ser–Ala–Arg–Lys–Leu⌐

⌐Leu–Gln–Asp–Ile–Met–Ser–Arg–Gln–Gln–Gly–Glu–Ser–Asn–Gln–Glu–Arg–Gly–Ala–Arg –Ala–Arg–Leu–NH₂

(a) Primary structure of growth hormone releasing hormone (GHRH)

Ala–Gly–Cys–Lys–Asn–Phe –Trp–Lys–Thr–Phe–Thr–Ser–Cys

(b) Primary structure of mammalian somatostatin (SS)

$$\underset{\text{O}}{\overset{\text{CO(CH}_2)_6\text{CH}_3}{|}}$$

Gly–Ser–Ser–Phe–Lys–Ser–Pro–Glu–His–Glu–Lys–Ala–Glu–Glu–Arg–Lys–Asp–Ser–Lys⌐

⌐Lys–Pro–Pro–Ala–Lys–Leu–Glu–Pro –Arg

(c) Primary structure of rat ghrelin

Fig 5.3. Amino acid sequences of growth hormone releasing hormone, somatostatin and ghrelin.

nucleus (PVN). The amino acid sequence of TRH is identical in porcine, ovine, bovine and human species. In addition, TRH induces PRL release in essentially all vertebrates studied.

The traditional concept of the regulation of GH release from the anterior pituitary primarily by hypothalamic stimulating (GHRH) and inhibiting (SS) factors has been modified by the discovery of an additional regulatory polypeptide. In the 1970s and 1980s, studies were carried out with synthetic polypeptides and non-peptides that induce GH release (GH secretagogues), with a goal of providing human diagnostic and treatment tools. These studies suggested that the synthetic secretagogues acted through a receptor distinct from the known GHRH receptor. This 'orphan' receptor, which had no known natural ligand, was called the GH secretagogue (GHS) receptor. Using a 'reverse pharmacology' approach, in which extracts from several organs were tested for their GHS receptor activity, it was found that the stomach was the major source of the natural GHS receptor ligand. This led to the isolation of a peptide by Japanese scientists in 1999 that was named ghrelin. The term ghrelin is derived from the Proto-Indo-European root 'ghre', for the word 'growth'. The suffix 'relin' means 'releasing substances'.

Ghrelin is a 28-amino acid polypeptide that was the first naturally occurring polypeptide to contain an octanoylated amino acid (ser-3). Ghrelin regulates energy expenditure, appetite as well as the GH axis. Ghrelin is produced by the pituitary and hypothalamus as well as mucosal enteroendocrine cells of the stomach. Ghrelin mRNA has also been found in descending concentrations in the small and large intestines, and in the pancreas, liver and kidney. Its secretion is induced by fasting and reduced by feeding. Ghrelin receptors are G-protein-linked receptors and are found in the hypothalamus, pituitary and various areas of the brain. Ghrelin acts through the hypothalamus and the pituitary to induce pituitary release of GH. The ghrelin mRNA and peptide in the anterior pituitary are increased by GHRH infusion and ghrelin may have a local autocrine or paracrine effect on stimulating GH release. In addition to the regulatory effects on GH, ghrelin has several direct physiological effects related to energy intake and utilization. Acting via neuropeptide Y (NPY) in the hypothalamus, ghrelin increases appetite, food intake and body weight gain. In addition, ghrelin has local effects in the gastrointestinal tract, where it stimulates gastric acid secretion and gastric motility. Thus, ghrelin provides an endocrine link between the stomach, hypothalamus and pituitary and coordinates the neuroendocrine regulation of energy balance with the GH/IGF-I system.

GH receptors

The GH receptor was the first member of the cytokine/haematopoietin receptor superfamily to be identified and cloned from human and rabbit liver in 1987. This receptor has now been cloned from laboratory rodents, cattle, sheep, swine and chickens. The GH receptors are classified as class I cytokine/haematopoietin receptors and also include the receptors for PRL, PL, leptin, erythropoietin, interleukins and the colony-stimulating factors (CSF) for immune cells. Class II cytokine receptors include those for the interferon-α/β, interferon-γ and interleukin-10.

There are three types of GH/PRL family of receptors that bind the GH- and PRL-related hormones to varying degrees and specificity in different species. The GH receptor is termed a somatogenic (growth-inducing) receptor. GH receptors are widespread and are found in most of the tissues of the body. The liver is an abundant source of the GH receptor, where it mediates the induction of IGF synthesis and secretion. GH receptors are also found in bone, cartilage, adipose tissue and skeletal muscle. The bGH receptor binds bovine, ovine and human GH with equal affinities, with a lower affinity for PRL and PL. The lactogenic receptor is found in many tissues, but is abundant in the mammary gland and liver. In the liver, the PRL receptor concentrations are present in higher concentrations in females than males, and are induced by oestrogens. This receptor binds PRL and PL with equal affinities that are higher than that of GH. The PL receptor of the placenta binds PL with greater affinity than PRL and PRL better than GH. The cross-reactivity of GH, PRL and PL with each other's receptors means that these hormones are capable of inducing growth and lactation. Although the primary function of GH is growth regulation and it is generally a weak promoter of milk synthesis, it is a strong inducer of lactogenesis in some species such as cattle. Likewise, the lactogenic effects of PRL and PL predominate, while these hormones have weak growth-promoting actions.

The GH receptor is a 120–130 kDa highly glycosylated protein, which consists of a single polypeptide chain (~620 amino acids, 70 kDa), containing a single transmembrane domain, without intrinsic kinase activity (Fig. 5.4). There are ten tyrosine (Y) residues in the cytoplasmic

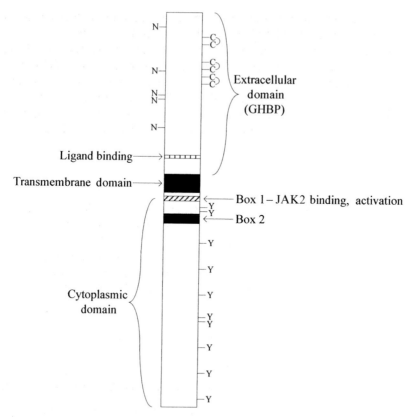

Fig. 5.4. The GH receptor, showing asparagine (N) sites for glycosylation, cysteines (C) that form intramolecular disulphide bonds, tyrosines available for phosphorylation and the Box 1 site for JAK2 binding.

domain of the GH receptor, some of which are phosphorylated by JAK. Multiple cysteines (C), forming disulphide bonds, are present in the extracellular domain. This domain is highly glycosylated on the numerous extracellular asparagines (N). After binding to GH, this receptor monomer forms a dimer with another monomeric GH receptor, binds JAK2 on the proline-rich Box 1 site of the cytoplasmic domain and activates the STAT transcription factors by tyrosine phosphorylation. The activation and signal transduction of the GH receptor via JAK has been discussed in Chapter 3.

Interestingly, the extracellular, ligand-binding domain of GH receptor is found in the circulation of all animals examined, including cattle, sheep, swine, horses, goats, cats and dogs. This truncated receptor acts as a GH-binding protein (GHBP) and is composed of roughly 246 amino acids that are identical to the extracellular domain of the GH receptor. It is produced primarily in the liver, where it is co-expressed with the GH receptor. The formation of the GHBP results from proteolytic cleavage of the GH receptor near the transmembrane site in rabbits and humans. In rodents, alternate splicing of the GH gene produces the GHBP. This soluble GH-binding entity is glycosylated, devoid of the transmembrane domain and the cytoplasmic transducer of the complete receptor. Circulating concentrations of GHBP are higher in females than males, increase with age and are correlated with body mass. It has been proposed that GHBP is an indicator of GH status and sensitivity. In addition, GHBP may regulate the activity of circulating GH by sequestering it, preventing its degradation and, thus, increasing its half-life in the circulation.

Metabolic actions of GH

GH is an anabolic hormone that affects most tissues. The effects of GH can be broadly divided into those which alter metabolism and those which promote growth of bone and skeletal muscle. These actions are, of course, overlapping, but it is convenient to examine the metabolic and growth effects separately. The metabolic effects of GH are wide-ranging and affect all three metabolic fuels: carbohydrates, proteins and fat (Table 5.1).

Table 5.1. Effects of growth hormone on metabolism of major nutrients.

Nutrient	GH effect
Proteins	Enhanced amino acid uptake and utilization (muscle)
	Enhanced protein synthesis, accretion (muscle)
	Reduced amino acid oxidation, catabolism (liver)
	Reduced blood urea nitrogen
	Reduced urinary nitrogen excretion
Carbohydrates	Increased glucose uptake (muscle)
	Reduced glucose uptake and oxidation (adipose)
	Increased gluconeogenesis/glycogenolysis (liver)
	Increased glucose release (liver)
	Reduced glucose clearance and catabolism
	Increased blood glucose
	Reduced insulin responsiveness
Lipids	Reduced lipogenesis (chronic, positive energy balance)
	Reduced insulin sensitivity
	Enhanced lipolysis (acute, negative energy balance)
	Reduced expression and activity of lipogenic enzymes

GH effects are species-specific. Humans will respond only to GH of human or primate origins. Before the production of GH from recombinant DNA, only GH from cadaver pituitaries could be used to treat GH-deficient humans and the use of purified GH to enhance animal production was unthinkable. GH from animals 'lower' on the evolutionary scale does not affect humans. Domestic animals respond best to GH from their own species. This is because of the diversity of protein hormones, which display different amino acid content between species. For example, the amino acid similarity between ovine and bGH is essentially identical (99.5%), while pGH is about 90% similar to bGH. In contrast, human GH has an amino acid similarity to bGH of only 68%. These differences in amino acid sequence between species are manifested in the binding to hepatic receptors from different species. Thus human GH is only one-tenth as effective in binding to the bGH receptor as is bGH. For this reason, bovine, ovine and pGH have no effects on humans.

Major target organs for GH are the liver, skeletal muscle, bone/cartilage and fat, but GH receptors are found in virtually all tissues. It is now known that most of GH effects on growth are mediated by IGF-I, which is induced at the local target tissue by GH. Within the tissues, IGFs, induced by GH, act primarily on a local level in autocrine and paracrine mechanisms. The effects of GH are often difficult to demonstrate *in vitro*, in the absence of IGF-I. This and other evidence suggests that many of the traditional or classical effects of GH seen when it is injected into animals are indirect and mediated by the IGF system (Fig. 5.5). The relationship between GH and the IGFs will be more fully elaborated after the following discussion of the effects of GH on nutrient metabolism.

The anabolic effects of GH on protein metabolism are seen at many levels. These effects can be detected in the whole animal and in individual organs, although many of these effects are probably indirect and due to direct effects of IGF-I. In general, when animals are treated with GH, this induces an overall positive nitrogen balance in the body. This is reflected by a reduction in circulating amino acids, decreased blood urea nitrogen concentrations and reduced urinary nitrogen excretion. This nitrogen-conserving effect of GH provides amino acids for increased muscle hypertrophy and muscle protein accretion in growing animals. In lactating animals, these amino acids are directed towards milk protein synthesis. GH treatment stimulates skeletal muscle and mammary gland amino acid uptake, reduces hepatic amino acid catabolism and increases protein synthesis *in vivo*. These effects are not seen in isolated muscle or mammary cells, suggesting that these effects of GH are indirect and mediated by IGF-I.

GH also plays a role in regulating carbohydrate metabolism. Along with glucagon, the glucocorticoids and the catecholamines, GH acts as an insulin counter-regulatory hormone to mobilize tissue stores of glucose to increase blood glucose levels. Treatment of lactating cows with GH reduces whole body glucose oxidation and increases the irreversible loss of glucose. GH has anti-insulin effects, inhibiting the actions of insulin on adipose glucose uptake. GH also blocks the inhibitory effects of insulin on hepatic gluconeo-

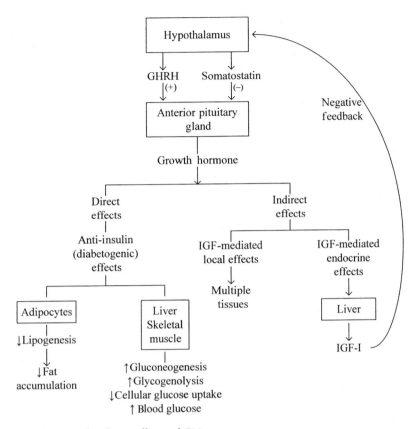

Fig. 5.5. The direct and indirect effects of GH.

genesis. In lactating cows, *de novo* synthesis of glucose via gluconeogenesis provides virtually all of the energy needed for milk synthesis. Liver stores of glycogen in these animals are inadequate to meet the needs for the energy required for milk synthesis. GH is also considered to be a diabetogenic hormone, increasing blood glucose and, in response to elevated glucose, circulating insulin concentrations. When given over long periods of time, GH can induce permanent diabetes, probably due to pancreatic islet cell 'burnout' in response to chronically elevated glucose. Hence, many of the effects of GH that result in an elevation of blood glucose are due to an inhibition of insulin-induced glucose utilization by the body, not to a direct stimulation of gluconeogenesis by GH.

GH treatment reduces lipid deposition. GH has effects on both lipogenesis and lipolysis, with the major effect on reducing lipogenesis, rather than increasing lipolysis. Although early studies reported lipolytic effects of GH, these have not been seen with highly purified recombinant GH used in experiments conducted since the 1990s. Effects of GH on lipid metabolism are chronic, seen over long periods of treatment *in vivo* and *in vitro*. GH effects on lipid metabolism are largely indirect, as GH acts by inhibiting insulin effects on adipose tissue glucose uptake via the cellular glucose transport protein, GLUT4, and subsequent glucose use for lipogenesis. GH treatment reduces the gene expression and activity of the key, rate-limiting lipogenic enzymes, FAS and ACC. In well-fed animals, lipolytic effects of GH are minor and GH treatment does not induce an increase in circulating free fatty acids and glycerol, products of lipolysis. However, if animals are in a negative energy balance, treatment with GH can induce lipolysis. This effect is transient and indirect. This is seen at the beginning of GH treatments of lactating dairy cattle, growing cattle and pigs, and is thought to be due to an increased lipolytic response to catecholamines, adrenal medullary hormones released in response to stress.

Excess and inadequate GH: giants and dwarfs

Excess or inadequate concentrations of GH lead to growth and metabolic anomalies with phenotypic and metabolic consequences. These are well characterized in humans and are representative of effects seen in animals with GH anomalies. The effects of excess GH depend upon the developmental stage in which the animal is exposed to GH. Excess GH secretion is usually seen as a result of an adenoma, an anterior pituitary gland tumour. When excessive GH is present prior to puberty, *gigantism* results. In this condition, the epiphyses of the long bones fuse at a later age than normal, resulting in excessive long bone growth and height. Constant exposure to GH in the growing animal also affects the visceral organs, resulting in splanchnomegaly, the enlargement of the liver, kidneys and the gastrointestinal tract. Skin and skeletal muscles also are hypertrophic under the influence of GH. Affected individuals suffer from diabetes due to the constant elevation of glucose, and subsequently insulin, under the influence of GH.

When adults are exposed to excess GH, a condition known as *acromegaly* results. This is characterized by growth of bones at the sites of existing cartilage and results in the enlargement of the extremities (feet, hands, nose, jaw) and a resultant 'coarsening' of features. These characteristics are due to the lateral overgrowth of bones after the epiphyses have fused. Other features of acromegaly include thyroid goitre, osteoarthritis, carpal tunnel syndrome and reproductive disorders.

Insufficient GH, as a result of hypopituitarism, leads to *dwarfism*. Hypopituitarism can result from a variety of causes, ranging from pituitary tumours, trauma to the pituitary, radiation exposure or genetics. Other than specific genetic defects in GH secretion or insensitivity, these hypopituitary syndromes are relatively non-specific and affect GH as well as the gonadotrophic hormones LH and FSH. As a result, most hypopituitary dwarfs are reproductively sterile and have infantile body proportions, with large heads and lack of secondary sex characteristics. More recently a syndrome called Laron dwarfism has been identified in humans. Affected individuals have normal levels of GH, but do not have the GH receptor, and are thus GH-resistant. A line of miniature Brahman cattle has been found to be the result of a mutation in the GH receptor, similar to the Laron dwarf syndrome in humans. As in the human syndrome, this animal is GH-insensitive and displays elevated circulating GH and reduced serum levels of IGF-I. Reduced growth rate and proportionally reduced adult body size have also been found in humans with mutations in the GHRH receptor, in which low circulating levels of GH and IGF-I are present as well as normal body proportions. In general, individuals affected with the classic hypopituitary dwarfism syndrome are phenotypically different from the small people called midgets. The latter condition is hereditary rather than hormonal and results in a smaller adult body form that is proportional to the conventional adult form. Midgets are fertile and possess all the attributes of normal-sized adults.

IGFs or Somatomedins

IGFs are small peptides which mediate many of the effects of GH. These growth factors play multiple roles in animal growth and development, acting as circulating hormones as well as growth factors that are produced in most, if not all, tissues that act via local autocrine and paracrine pathways. Their actions encompass insulin-like effects on metabolism, GH-like effects on animal growth and effects on cell division and differentiation in tissues derived from embryonic mesoderm.

Discovery of the IGFs

In 1957, Salmon and Daughaday published the first evidence for serum factors which had direct effects on cartilage growth. These scientists were studying the effects of serum on the incorporation of radioactive sulphur into chondroitin sulphate of rat cartilage *in vitro*, with a focus on GH effects. They found that serum from normal rats stimulated sulphate incorporation while serum from hypophysectomized rats had no effect. This suggested that GH was stimulating cartilage growth. However, when GH was added to the hypophysectomized rat serum there was no effect on sulphate incorporation. When injected into hypophysectomized rats, GH treatment induced a positive growth response. These observations suggested that GH did not have a direct effect on cartilage growth and that the effects of GH were mediated by a circulating factor not produced by the pituitary. This was the first evidence for the existence of a *sulphation factor* which mediated GH effects. Dr Daughaday later named this *somatomedin*, a factor which mediates the effects of ST, or GH. The somatomedin fraction was later separated into two different sub-fractions, somatomedin C, whose serum concentration was GH-dependent, and somatomedin A, which was not.

The initial observations of Daughaday's group languished until 1963, when Swiss scientists (Froesch, Rinderknecht, Humbel) were examining the paradoxical findings that serum had insulin-like effects on increasing glucose uptake in skeletal muscle and fat cells which were much greater than expected from insulin alone. These conclusions were due to the observation that antibodies to insulin did not suppress these insulin effects. This group called this activity *non-suppressible insulin-like activity* (NSILA). After isolation and separation of the NSILA activity into two distinct fractions, this activity was renamed IGF-I and IGF-II.

In 1972, Pierson and Temin were investigating low molecular weight serum factors which stimulated cell growth *in vitro*. They succeeded in isolating mitogenic peptides from serum with estimated molecular weights less than 10 kDa. As a result of the mitogenic effects of these peptides, Pierson and Temin called this activity *multiplication-stimulating activity* (MSA). Further studies by Temin's group showed that the liver was the source of MSA. It is now known that the original MSA is equivalent to IGF-II.

These studies established the IGFs as versatile molecules which display the dual characteristics of serum-borne endocrine hormones and mitosis-inducing growth factors. The IGFs have effects on cartilage growth, stimulate mitosis in many cells and have both insulin-like and GH-like effects. These studies led to the formulation of the somatomedin hypothesis (Fig. 5.6). This hypothesis states that the effects of GH on target tissues are not direct, but are mediated by IGFs synthesized and secreted by the liver under the control of GH. The promulgation of this hypothesis, in the early 1980s, altered fundamentally the field of endocrinology. The discovery and characterization of the biology of the IGFs demonstrated, for the first time, that a traditional organ of metabolism, the liver, also acted as an endocrine organ that secreted IGFs into the circulation. It also relegated GH to the status of an inducing factor that had few, if any, direct effects on organs other than the

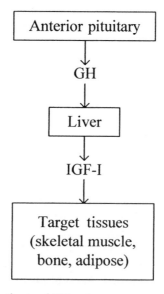

Fig. 5.6. The somatomedin hypothesis of GH action.

liver. In the ensuing years, it has been shown that GH has both direct and indirect effects on some tissues and that the role of endocrine IGF is less than that of IGF produced locally under the stimulation of GH. Modifications and extensions of the somatomedin hypothesis will be discussed later in this chapter.

IGF genes and molecules

Although the mature IGF peptides contain at most 70 amino acids and could be coded for by 210 bases, the IGF genes are very large and complex. The IGF-I gene consists of at least six exons separated by five introns and covers more than 80 kb of DNA. The IGF-II gene consists of nine exons and spans about 30 kb of DNA. Several different IGF mRNA species arise from transcription of the genes due to alternative splicing, polyadenylation and multiple promoter sites. Some transcripts are specific to different organs and tissues and may play important roles in tissue development and embryonic growth and differentiation.

The two types of IGF, IGF-I and IGF-II, are distinguished by their biochemical and biological characteristics. IGF-I is considered to be the primary biologically active IGF in adult mammals and is secreted in an endocrine fashion by the liver in response to GH. IGF-I was originally dubbed somatomedin C by Daughaday and is produced not only by the liver, but also by many other tissues. IGF-I has a basic isoelectric point (pI) of about 7.8 and consists of 70 amino acids in all mammals studied. IGF-I is thought to mediate many of the effects of GH and is important for late fetal growth and initiating early postnatal growth. IGF-II (identical to somatomedin A and MSA) is a polypeptide with a neutral pI of about 7.0 and consists of 66 or 67 amino acids in mammals. It is secreted independently of GH and is thought to be important in the regulation of early fetal growth.

The IGFs have a molecular structure that is very similar to proinsulin, the precursor to insulin (Fig. 5.7). Both IGF-I and IGF-II consist of a single polypeptide chain with molecular weights of about 7500 Da. Like proinsulin, the IGF polypeptides contain two disulphide bonds to maintain the tertiary structure and consist of three functional domains (A, B, C). When the inactive proinsulin is converted to active insulin, the C domain (C-peptide) is enzymatically removed, resulting in an active insulin molecule with two peptide subunits held together by disulphide bonds. Unlike insulin, the C-peptide is not cleaved in IGFs. The A and B domains of the IGFs are about 45% identical to insulin. The C domain consists of 31 to 35 amino acids in proinsulin, 12 in IGF-I and eight in IGF-II. The sequence of the IGF-I and IGF-II molecules is highly conserved between different mammalian species. The IGF-I peptide is identical in humans, swine and cattle, with a single amino acid change in ovine IGF-I, three for rats and four in mice. Bovine and human IGF-II differ from one another by three amino acids, while rat and mouse IGF-II differ from the human molecule by four and six amino acids, respectively.

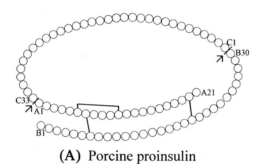

(A) Porcine proinsulin

(B) Human IGF-I

Fig. 5.7. The primary structures of (A) porcine proinsulin and (B) human IGF-I. The amino acids in black circles of the IGF-I structure are identical in both human insulin and IGF-I.

IGF receptors

The effects of the IGFs are mediated by three receptors which bind IGFs, the insulin receptor, the Type I IGF receptor and the Type II IGF receptor (Fig. 5.8). The overlapping biological effects of the IGFs and insulin are reflected not only by the overall gross similarity of these molecules, but also by the overlapping molecular identity and cross-reactivity of ligand binding by the insulin and IGF-I receptors. The insulin and Type I IGF receptors are very similar in overall structure and their amino acid sequences are about 30% identical. These large molecules (~450 kDa) are heterotetramers, consisting of two identical extracellular ligand-binding α subunits and two β subunits containing the transmembrane and cytoplasmic domains. The cytoplasmic β subunits of the insulin and Type I IGF receptors are TK which catalyse the phosphorylation of intracellular second messengers. These receptors were discussed in detail in Chapter 3.

In contrast, the third receptor for IGFs, the Type II IGF receptor, consists of a single glycoprotein chain, with a molecular weight of ~250 kDa. This molecule is also known as the cation-independent mannose-6-phosphate (M-6-P) receptor. The plasma membrane form of this receptor consists primarily of an extracellular domain that consists of 15 repeats of approximately 147 amino acids. The extracellular domain has two binding sites for M-6-P and a single IGF-II binding site. The Type II receptor is embedded in the plasma

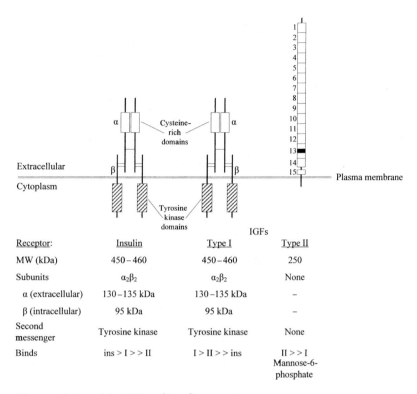

Fig. 5.8. Characteristics of the IGF and insulin receptors.

Receptor:	Insulin	Type I	Type II
MW (kDa)	450–460	450–460	250
Subunits	$\alpha_2\beta_2$	$\alpha_2\beta_2$	None
α (extracellular)	130–135 kDa	130–135 kDa	–
β (intracellular)	95 kDa	95 kDa	–
Second messenger	Tyrosine kinase	Tyrosine kinase	None
Binds	ins > I > > II	I > II > > ins	II > > I Mannose-6-phosphate

membrane by its transmembrane domain, but has only a truncated cytoplasmic tail. It is the primary cell surface binding entity for IGF-II. IGF-I, but not insulin, also binds slightly to this receptor. The Type II IGF receptor has no known kinase activity or associated second messenger system. For this reason, it is not believed to function as a hormone receptor. It is located primarily within the intracellular membranes of the cytoplasm where it binds lysosomal enzymes via their M-6-P residues. The primary biological function of the IGF-II/M-6-P receptor is believed to be in transporting hydrolytic enzymes from the Golgi apparatus to the lysosomes, where they are involved in cellular catabolism of specific substrates. In addition, the Type II IGF receptor is involved in the clearance and catabolism of circulating IGF-II. The plasma membrane form of this receptor is rapidly internalized and IGF-II bound to the receptor is degraded in lysosomes. The internalization and breakdown of IGF-II prevent development of excessive levels of IGF-II, which can be detrimental to the animal, especially during embryonic development. Knockout mice in which the Type II receptor is deleted exhibit elevated IGF-II concentrations, enlarged viscera and rarely live beyond birth. These effects are believed to be a result of exposure to excessive IGF-II, which results as a consequence of the absence of degradation by the Type II receptor. The biological effects of IGF-II are mediated through the IGF-I receptor.

IGF-binding proteins

The adult, circulating concentrations of the IGFs are quite high for a hormone, generally above 100 ng/ml (13 nmol/l). Cellular responses to IGF-I are induced at much lower levels, in the order of 10 to 20 ng/ml. The potential effects of excess serum concentrations of the IGFs are dampened by the binding and sequestration of IGFs by serum binding proteins. Roughly 99% of circulating IGFs are bound to binding proteins. In addition, many tissues produce the IGFBPs locally. These binding proteins reversibly bind IGF-I and IGF-II to high affinity, non-covalent binding sites. The affinity of IGFBP for IGFs is 10 to 40 times higher than the IGF-I receptor, effectively removing IGFBP-bound IGF from interactions with its target tissue receptors.

There are six IGFBPs, numbered 1 to 6. Most of the IGFBPs have equal affinities for IGF-I and IGF-II, but IGFBP-6 binds IGF-II with a 20- to 70-fold higher affinity than IGF-I. The major serum IGFBPs were discovered when IGF activity was isolated in the high molecular weight fractions after size exclusion chromatography of serum. These early studies showed that a majority of IGF activity was associated with the 40 and 150 kDa molecular weight fractions, with 70–80% of the IGF activity in the high molecular weight, 150 kDa fraction. This high molecular weight binding protein was named IGFBP-3. GH stimulates the hepatic secretion of this glycoprotein. IGFBP-3 consists of an acid-stable subunit (40–45 kDa), which binds IGF, and an acid-labile subunit (85 kDa). The second major serum-binding protein is IGFBP-2. This IGFBP accounted for the other 20% to 30% of bound serum IGF, originally designated as the 40 kDa fraction. It is now known that IGFBP-2 is a 31.3 kDa protein that is also secreted by the liver. The other IGFBPs are single-chain proteins, of roughly 25 kDa. These include IGFBP-1, a placental protein found mainly in fetal amniotic fluid. IGFBP-4 is widespread and found in serum, seminal plasma, fibroblasts and osteoblasts. IGFBP-5 and IGFBP-6 are less abundant binding proteins found in serum and tissues.

In general, circulating IGF bound to IGFBP is unavailable for receptor binding and is not biologically active. The regulation of IGF actions is related to the interactions of IGF with binding proteins in the serum and at the tissue level. The IGFBPs are thought to regulate IGF action in a number of ways. As the binding is reversible and in chemical equilibrium with nonbound (free) IGF, the IGF–IGFBP complex provides a constant source of additional IGF. As free IGF levels are reduced by IGF use and metabolism, it is replaced by the release of IGF from the IGFBP. In addition, IGFBP-bound IGF has a longer half-life than unbound, or free, IGF. Thus, binding to IGFBP increases the circulating half-life of IGF, probably by reducing IGF degradation.

In contrast to the primarily inhibitory effects of IGFBP on IGF activity, three IGFBPs increase the activity of IGFs: IGFBP-1, -3, and -5. This enhancement of IGF activity is attributed to different mechanisms. Phosphorylation of the IGFBP-1 molecule increases its affinity for IGF by sixfold and the lower affinity of dephosphorylated IGFBP-1 induces the release of bound

IGF. This enhances the effect of IGF on DNA synthesis in some cells. This increased IGF activity is thought to be due to a shift of the binding of IGF from the lower affinity, dephosphorylated IGFBP to the higher affinity IGF-I receptor. IGFBP-3 binds to cell surfaces while IGFBP-5 is associated with the ECM. The binding to cell membranes and matrix proteins reduces the affinity of IGFBP-3 and -5 for IGF, resulting in the release of IGFs, which stimulate tissue receptors. Local production of IGFBP may also protect IGFs from proteolytic degradation, provide a local tissue reservoir of IGF, and present IGF to local tissue receptors. IGFBP-1 and -2 have an Arg-Gly-Asp (RGD) sequence which binds to specific surface-bound integrin receptors. In general, the actions of the IGFBP are likely to play a more pronounced regulatory role in the localized actions of IGF.

From a practical standpoint, the measurement of IGFs using competitive binding methods, such as radioimmunoassay or radioreceptor assay, are greatly influenced by the presence of the IGFBPs. Whether the biologically relevant portion of the IGFs is the total (free and IGFBP-bound) IGF or the free (non-bound) IGF, the measurement of IGFs cannot be accomplished in the presence of the IGFBPs, due to the IGFBP competition for binding sites on the immunoglobulins or receptors used for analysis. The IGFBPs can be removed physically, using size exclusion chromatography to separate the high molecular weight IGFBPs from the smaller IGFs. Analysis of the low molecular weight fraction provides a measure of free IGF and is likely the most relevant measure. This method is cumbersome, expensive and time-consuming. The majority of reports of IGF concentrations use a chemical denaturation method, by treatment of serum with acid or acid–ethanol. This removes the IGFBPs and releases IGFs for analysis, providing a measure of total IGF. As IGFBP types and affinities vary with species, developmental stage (fetal, neonatal and adult) and physiological state (e.g. pregnant vs non-pregnant), methods to remove these binding proteins must be validated for each application.

Metabolic effects of the IGFs

Adult serum levels of IGF-I are very high for a hormone, about 100 to 150 ng/ml, while those of IGF-II are about threefold higher. The liver produces about 90% of the IGF-I in the circulation and, until recently, IGF-I was thought to act in a traditional endocrine manner. High serum IGF-I levels act in a negative feedback loop at the hypothalamus, inducing SS release and, hence, reducing GH secretion. Additional IGF is produced in most, if not all, tissues, where it acts in an autocrine and/or paracrine manner, affecting local tissues without the intervention of the circulation. Recent data, discussed below, suggest that local tissue production of IGF-I is more important in regulating animal growth than is endocrine IGF-I.

The IGFs have primary effects as mitogenic and differentiation-inducing growth factors and secondarily as insulin-like factors. The mitogenic effects of the IGFs are quite pronounced and the IGFs are active at low nanomolar concentrations. Treatment of cells with IGF stimulates RNA and DNA synthesis in many cells with a mesodermal origin. In addition, IGFs increase amino acid uptake, inhibit protein degradation and stimulate protein synthesis in many tissues. In cartilage, IGFs increase collagen and proteoglycan synthesis. In fat cells, the IGFs stimulate lipid synthesis and reduce lipolysis, effects opposite to those of GH. Specific effects of the IGFs will be discussed in the following chapters on muscle, fat and bone growth and development.

As we have seen, IGFs cross-react with the insulin receptor at higher pharmacological concentrations. At higher concentrations, the IGFs can have insulin-like effects. IGF-I is about 1/100 to 1/5 as potent as insulin in inducing insulin-like effects, probably via interactions with the insulin receptor. For example, high doses of IGF-I induce increased glucose transport and oxidation by adipose tissue. In addition, at high concentrations, IGF-I can induce transient hypoglycaemia, accompanied by increased glycogen synthesis in liver and muscle. Overall, these insulin-like effects of the IGFs induce anabolic metabolism in target tissues, leading to a net increase of glycogen, protein and lipid deposition. Interestingly, when present in pharmacological doses, insulin can act as a mitogen, a process presumably mediated by the IGF-I receptor.

Effects of the IGFs on animal growth

The IGFs have many effects on animal growth. Early observations showed that, in the growing animal, IGF levels increase with postnatal age. IGF-I serum concentrations in the neonatal animal are relatively low, but gradually increase during maturation, reach a peak at the time of puberty and then gradually decline throughout adulthood. Several studies have shown that serum levels of IGF-I are proportional to birth weight and to adult body weight. In many species, including humans, livestock and companion animals, IGF-I concentrations are proportional to body size. In dogs, for example, IGF-I concentrations increase with breed sizes, from miniature to toy to standard-sized poodles (Table 5.2).

Similar observations have been made in other species, including swine, cattle and sheep. The relatively constant circulating levels of IGF-I, propor-

Table 5.2. Correlation of plasma IGF-I concentrations and adult body size of dogs.

Poodle breed	Weight (kg)	IGF-I (ng/ml)
Toy	3.0±0.2	16±4
Miniature	6.2±0.4	24±5
Standard	20.9±1.6	96±15

From Eigenmann *et al.* (1984).

tional to GH concentrations, are much easier to measure than GH, and provide an excellent measure of the growth and GH status of animals. When
IGF-I is injected into hypophysectomized or normal animals, growth rates
are increased (Fig. 5.9). Transgenic IGF-I mice, which express excess IGF-I,
have higher growth rates than normal mice, but have a disproportionate
increase in the sizes of brain, pancreas, kidney, spleen and thymus. In general, IGF-I is not as potent as GH in growth induction and does not mimic all
effects of GH.

Fetal and early neonatal growth in most species is independent of GH.
Animals without a pituitary gland, GH or the GH receptor develop normally
and have expected birth weights. In the mammalian fetus, circulating concentrations of GH are relatively high, but the fetal liver has little or no GH
receptor, and IGF secretion is independent of GH. In the fetal sheep liver, for
example, GH receptors are undetectable, but the fetus has abundant receptors for PRL and low levels of PL receptor. Binding to hepatic GH receptors
increases rapidly in the newborn lamb, and as GH binding increases, there
is a proportional increase in postnatal serum IGF-I levels, suggesting that the
appearance of hepatic GH receptors is functional and mediates the induction
of IGF-I secretion that stimulates postnatal growth. In calves, there is no
detectable GH binding to liver receptors up to the second day postpartum.
Significant GH binding is not seen until 3 weeks postpartum, and increases
up until 12 weeks.

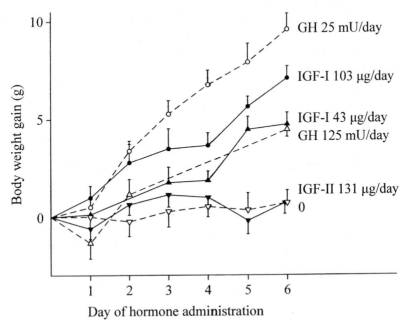

Fig. 5.9. Effects of GH and IGF injections on growth of hypophysectomized rats. (With
permission from Schoenle *et al.*, 1985.)

The effects of removing the influence of IGF-I and IGF-II on fetal and postnatal growth have been explored in 'knockout' mice that have had the IGF-I or -II gene deleted. When the IGF-I gene is deleted, the majority of animals die immediately after birth due to the lack of skeletal muscle, and hence diaphragm, development. Surviving animals are stunted, weighing only 60% of normal birth weight and at adulthood are only 30% of the normal body weights. This suggests that IGF-I plays a major role in fetal as well as postnatal growth. Treatment of growing, IGF-I-deficient mice with GH does not improve growth, suggesting that the presence of IGF-I, either local or endocrine, is required for the growth-promoting effects of GH. When the IGF-II gene is deleted, most animals are viable, but are only 60% of normal birth weight and adult body weight. Thus, the major role of IGF-II is during fetal development, with minimal or no effects on postnatal development. Most of the IGF-II effects during fetal development are indirect, due to effects on placental growth. The IGF-II knockout mice have reductions in placental weights that are proportional to the reduction of birth weights.

Recent studies have examined the role of endocrine vs paracrine and autocrine effects of IGF-I on animal growth. In these experiments, the hepatic IGF-I gene is selectively deleted. This removes the endocrine source of IGF-I without affecting local tissue production of IGF-I. In these animals, only extrahepatic, locally produced IGF-I is present. In the non-selective IGF knockout mice described above, the IGF genes are inactive in all tissues and throughout fetal, neonatal and adult development. The selective deletion of hepatic IGF-I gene occurs in the late fetal stages of development. Hence, the IGF-I effects on fetal growth are largely eliminated.

In the animals that lack the hepatic IGF-I gene, circulating IGF-I is reduced by 75% or more, while GH concentrations are elevated fourfold. This indicates that endocrine IGF-I is important in the negative feedback control of GH secretion, as the lower circulating levels of IGF-I are believed to relieve the normal GH inhibition by IGF-I. Surprisingly, the growth of these animals, as reflected by femoral bone and body length and organ mass, was not altered. In addition, sexual maturation and lactation were normal. Messenger RNA concentrations for IGF-I in heart, skeletal muscle, fat, spleen and kidney were unaltered, suggesting that IGF-I gene expression was not increased in the absence of circulating IGF-I or the presence of excess GH. The lack of a GH effect on tissue levels of IGF-I mRNA in these mice has been ascribed to the observation that GH is no longer released in a pulsatile fashion, which may be needed for mRNA induction. Likewise, there was no change in the concentrations of tissue IGF-I receptor mRNA.

In sum, these studies with targeted deletion of the liver IGF-I gene have demonstrated that circulating endocrine IGF-I is not involved in the regulation of postnatal growth. Locally produced IGF-I is the major regulator of postnatal growth. The control of local IGF-I synthesis and secretion is, in many cases, dependent upon GH stimulation and GH can have direct as well as indirect effects (through local IGF-I production) in stimulating the growth of adipose tissue, bone and skeletal muscle.

Modification of the somatomedin hypothesis

The original somatomedin hypothesis posited that most, if not all, effects of GH were mediated by endocrine IGF, produced by the liver under GH stimulation. This hypothesis was formulated before it was shown, in 1980, that IGF mRNA was present in virtually all fetal, neonatal and adult tissues. The validity of the somatomedin hypothesis was tested by Isaakson in 1982. To examine the direct effects of GH on longitudinal bone growth, in the absence of liver production of IGF-I, GH was injected directly into the tibial growth plate of hypophysectomized rats. This stimulated bone growth in the injected, but not the uninjected tibia, suggesting that GH had a direct effect on bone growth and that endocrine IGF from the liver was not involved. However, when antiserum to IGF-I was injected with GH (to inhibit the effects of local IGF-I) no bone growth was observed. These studies showed that the GH effects on bone growth were indeed indirect, but were not mediated by endocrine IGF-I. Instead, GH stimulated the production of local, bone-derived IGF-I, which acted in a paracrine or autocrine manner to induce tissue growth.

These observations, and similar ones by Green using adipose tissue, led to the formulation of the dual effector hypothesis for GH/IGF-I effects on tissue growth and differentiation (Fig. 5.10). This hypothesis proposes that GH

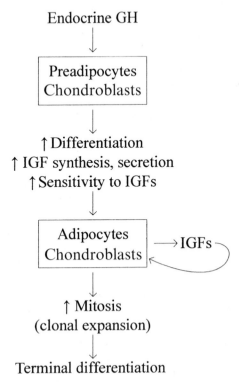

Fig. 5.10. The dual effector hypothesis of GH and IGF-I action.

stimulates the initial differentiation of adipocyte and chondrocyte precursor cells. This results in two events: the development of IGF-I responsiveness and the expression of the IGF-I gene. IGF-I, in turn, is secreted locally and it acts to stimulate mitosis and clonal expansion of adipocytes and chondrocytes, acting in a local, autocrine or paracrine fashion. Amplified cell populations then undergo final maturation. This modification of the somatomedin hypothesis accounts for the dual roles of GH and IGF-I on the growth and differentiation of cartilage and adipose tissue. Together with the observations discussed earlier in mice with selective deletion of the hepatic IGF-I gene, and the emphasis on autocrine and paracrine actions of IGF-I, the original somatomedin hypothesis must be reconsidered. With the exception of the negative feedback control of GH secretion, the major effects of the IGFs on growth and development are likely not to be endocrine in nature. Although these effects are stimulated by treatment with either GH or the IGFs, they are mediated by the IGFs in a local, tissue-specific manner via autocrine and paracrine mechanisms (Fig. 5.11).

Effects of GH on Farm Animal Production

The observations that the GH/IGF-I system enhanced muscle deposition and reduced fat content, coupled with the relatively new science of recombinant DNA for production of large quantities of these proteins, led to several trials of GH (called bST by Monsanto) on animal production systems beginning in the early 1980s. Monsanto was the first company to put a large

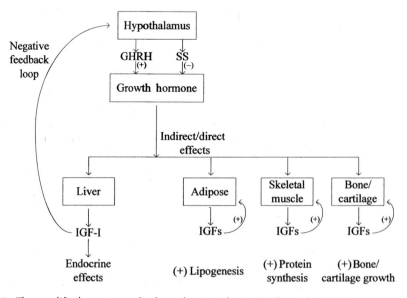

Fig. 5.11. The modified somatomedin hypothesis. (After LeRoith *et al.*, 2001.)

effort and investment into the production and use of GH to enhance animal production. As with the β-agonists, the major effects of GH in enhancing farm animal production result from nutrient repartitioning, by directing nutrient energy away from fat deposition and toward milk or muscle protein synthesis.

The primary focus for the commercial use of GH in animal production is in dairy cattle. The commercial use of bST in the USA began in 1994 and GH is now used in more than 2 million dairy cattle in 25 countries. The European Union prohibits its use. GH is given during the last 80% of lactation and increases milk yield by 10–15%. GH has no effects on milk composition, including protein, lactose, fat and minerals/vitamins. GH and IGF-I concentrations in milk are unaffected. As with all growth promotants, GH-treated animals require increased nutrients, primarily in the form of protein and amino acid supplements, which provide the needed energy and amino acid precursors for increased milk production. The increase in milk production efficiency offsets the added costs of feed supplementation.

The chemical instability of the GH molecule makes GH treatment of animals a problem. As GH is a protein, it is digested with other dietary proteins in the gastrointestinal tract. This makes the oral administration of GH impossible. Like most proteins, GH is susceptible to oxidation and denaturation, especially when in dilute aqueous solutions. Thus, injectable GH must be kept refrigerated when not in use and, in early trials, daily injections of GH were administered. Relatively long-lasting implants containing 500 mg of GH have now been developed and marketed for use in dairy cattle, but these must be replaced at 2-week intervals. This makes the administration of GH labour-intensive and amenable only to intensive production systems such as the dairy industry.

Studies on the effects of GH on the growth performance of cattle have proven disappointing. The effects of GH in these animals are small and inconsistent. Daily injections or weekly implants of GH into finishing steers or heifers over 3-month periods demonstrated dose-dependent increases in ADG and feed efficiency, while reducing feed intake. In steers, GH injected daily at 16.5 to 33 μg/kg body weight/day increased ADG by about 10% and feed efficiency by 10% to 20%, and reduced feed intake by 2% to 5%. Higher doses of GH (100 μg/kg/day) affected only feed efficiency, while 300 μg/kg/day reduced gain, intake and efficiency. For comparison, anabolic steroid implants containing oestradiol benzoate and trenbolone acetate (TBA) induced an increase of about 30% in ADG and a 20% to 35% in feed efficiency while reducing feed intake to be about 5%. Small or no effects of GH treatment on final body weights, carcass weight, loin eye area or backfat thickness have been reported. Effects of GH in meat ruminants are limited by lack of adequate nutrition, especially available amino acids. Animals must receive diets which are higher in rumenal escape protein, essential amino acids and energy to support the increased protein accretion rates and intake induced by GH. Even in studies in which these energy sources are provided, the effects on ruminant growth are minimal. As a result, GH has not been adopted in beef cattle production systems.

In contrast to the minimal effects of GH in beef cattle, the effects of GH on the growth and body composition of swine are dramatic. Treatment of pigs with GH induces large increases in feed efficiency (with reduced feed intake), ADG, carcass protein and lean carcass components and reduces body fat in a dose-dependent manner (Fig. 5.12).

Many experiments with growing pigs have shown that when GH was injected at 100 µg/kg body weight/day, ADG increased by 10% to 20%, feed intake was reduced by 15% and feed efficiency increased by 13% to 33%. At the same time, lipid accretion was reduced by up to 79% and protein deposition was increased by up to 62%. It is possible that these tremendous effects on body composition and nutrient partitioning from fat to muscle deposition from GH treatment may be mediated by the IGFs. A study that looked at the

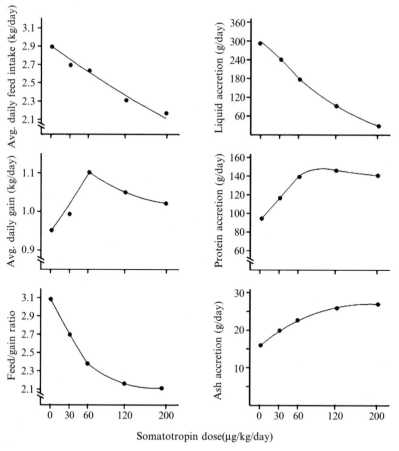

Fig. 5.12. Dose–response effects of GH in growing swine. (With permission from Campion et al., 1989. *Animal Growth Regulation,* Plenum Press.)

effects of IGF-I or GH treatment, alone or in combination, of pre-pubertal barrows has been done. The results of this study are shown in Table 5.3.

In this study, which used optimal doses of GH, treatment with GH or IGF-I did not alter feed intake. All treatments increased ADG and slaughter weight, but the effects of GH were much greater than those of IGF-I. GH had a large positive effect on feed efficiency, while IGF-I treatment did not affect feed efficiency. While IGF-I stimulated a 33% increase in carcass protein, the GH treatment induced an 88% increase in carcass protein. Only a small increase in lean cuts was induced by IGF-I, while GH treatment resulted in a 16% increase. IGF-I increased perirenal fat, carcass fat, kidney and pancreas weights. All vital organ weights (heart, lung, liver, kidney, spleen) were increased by GH treatment. The combined treatment of GH and IGF-I resulted in effects that were not different from GH given alone. This study suggested that treatment of growing barrows with GH induced significant positive effects on swine growth production characteristics. GH was much more effective than IGF-I in increasing lean body mass and protein deposition, while the effects of IGF-I were minimal. In these animals, it appears that the effects of GH were not mediated by endocrine IGF-I and were likely due to direct effects of GH. The local production and stimulation of tissues by autocrine/paracrine IGF-I, under GH control, may play a role in the observed effects of GH.

GH and the development of transgenic animals

The GH gene was the first to be used to develop a transgenic animal that overexpressed the product of a gene foreign to the natural genome of a mammal. In 1982, Ralph Brinster's group at the University of Pennsylvania combined the bGH gene and the mouse metallothionein-I promoter in a bacterial plasmid (Palmiter et al., (1982)). The metallothionein promoter allowed the induction of the GH gene in response to the metals zinc or cadmium. This recombinant DNA was then injected into the pronuclei of mouse eggs where it inserted itself into the mouse DNA. Roughly 600 copies of this gene were injected into each egg. A total of 170 resulting eggs were transferred into foster mothers and allowed to come to term. Of the 170 transferred eggs,

Table 5.3. Effects of IGF-I or GH treatment, alone or in combination, in swine (%).

Treatment (dose)	ADG	FE	Carc. prot.	Lean cuts
IGF-I (2 × 33 µg/kg/day)	+22	n.s.	+33	+5
pGH (33 µg/kg/day)	+43	+60	+88	+16
IGF-I + pGH (33+33)	Same as GH alone			

Adapted from Klindt et al. (1998).

21 animals developed to term and survived parturition. Seven of the surviving animals were positive for the presence of the GH–metallothionein construct. Breeding studies showed that only one mouse was capable of transmitting the gene in a Mendelian manner to its offspring.

Postnatal growth of the transgenic mice was proportional to the number of copies of the GH gene present in the tissues and to the expression of GH mRNA. There was a great deal of individual variation in the incorporation of the GH gene and tissue expression of GH mRNA. The serum concentrations of GH in four of the seven transgenic mice were 100–800 times greater than in control littermates and body weights were up to double those of control, non-transgenic littermates. Gigantism was observed in the transgenic mice and females were infertile. The animals' livers were enlarged and many had hepatic lesions. In addition, the animals were insulin-resistant, displaying the characteristics of Type II diabetes.

This pioneering study demonstrated that a foreign gene could be successfully transferred into a mammal. Unfortunately, there were many problems with these transgenics. For example, the GH gene is normally expressed only in specific cells of the anterior pituitary, and in the transgenic animal GH is incorporated and expressed by all tissues of the animal. This can lead to high local concentrations of GH in tissues that are not usually exposed to this extreme of GH concentration. Expression of the gene was largely unregulated, despite the presence of the metallothionein gene, and massive pharmacological levels of circulating GH were observed in the transgenic animals. The expression and function of GH in mammals is regulated by nutrients and developmental stage, while the regulation of GH expression in the transgenic mice was uncontrolled by development or nutrition. This study showed that the regulation of foreign gene expression in animals needed to be regulated to avoid constant, high levels of the gene product at the organ and systemic level. A regulatory system that controls gene expression in a manner similar to that of the natural gene is required to reap the benefits of transgenic animals.

A study was reported in 1990 by Richard Hanson's group at Case Western Reserve University (McGrane et al., (1990)) that was designed to overcome the problems seen with the unregulated expression of GH in the GH/MT-I transgenic mice. This group spliced bGH gene to the promoter for the hepatic enzyme phosphoenolpyruvate carboxykinase (PEPCK). This gene is expressed in a tissue-specific manner, and is controlled by nutrients, hormones and the developmental stage of the animals. By combining this promoter with the GH gene, it was hypothesized that a more controlled expression of the transgenic gene could be attained.

PEPCK catalyses the first step in hepatic gluconeogenesis, the synthesis of glucose from non-carbohydrate sources. PEPCK activity is localized to the adult liver, kidney and small intestine, but some activity is also detectable in the mammary gland, fat and skeletal muscle. The mammalian fetus receives all of its glucose by placental transfer from maternal sources. Therefore, the PEPCK gene is not expressed in the fetus, as there is no requirement for endogenous glucose synthesis. During fetal development, elevated insulin and glucose levels inhibit expression of the PEPCK gene. At birth, when the connection to maternal sources of glucose is severed and gluconeogenesis becomes important, the PEPCK gene is turned on. This occurs when neonatal levels of insulin and glucose drop and the concentrations of glucagon and glucocorticoid (cortisol) increase.

The PEPCK promoter region contains several response elements that regulate the expression of the PEPCK gene (Fig. 5.13). The promoter contains an insulin response element (IRE). Insulin inhibits PEPCK expression via the TK cascade, which activates a transcription factor that negatively regulates the PEPCK gene. A glucocorticoid response element (GRE) and a thyroid hormone response element (TRE) on the PEPCK gene promoter respond to the respective nuclear receptors, which act as transcription factors, for these hormones. Glucagon stimulates the PEPCK gene via the cAMP cascade and the cAMP response element-binding protein (CREBP) that binds to the CREI sequence. Tissue specificity of the PEPCK gene expression is conferred by the P2 site, which binds hepatic nuclear factor-1. In addition, promoter-binding sites for C/EBP and TFIID (transcription factor IID) are also present in the PEPCK promoter region.

In transgenic mice, expression of the PEPCK/bGH gene was limited to a specific area of the liver, the periportal hepatic cells. Its expression was also regulated developmentally. The PEPCK promoter-driven GH gene was inactive in the fetus, but expressed in the neonatal and adult animal. The expression of GH was repressed by postprandial elevations of insulin and glucose inhibited GH secretion in the transgenic mice. Gene expression of GH in the PEPCK/bGH transgenic mice was induced by glucagon and cortisol. Generation of transgenic animals with a promoter region that responds in a relatively physiological manner to changes in hormones, nutrients and developmental stage illustrates the complexity of the control of gene expression and provides an animal in which the gene is more closely regulated in a tissue-, developmental and nutrient-dependent manner.

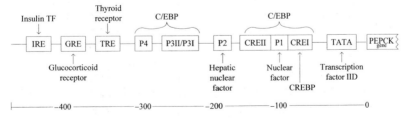

Fig. 5.13. The promoter region of the PEPCK gene. The lower scale indicates the number of base pairs of the promoter region preceding the PEPCK gene.

References and Further Reading

Dalke, B.S., Roeder, R.A., Kasser, T.R., Veenhuizen, J.J., Hunt, C.W., Hinman, D.D. and Schelling, G.T. (1992) Dose–response effects of recombinant bovine somatotropin implants on feedlot performance in steers. *Journal of Animal Science* 70, 2130–2137.

Eigenmann, J.E., Patterson, D.F. and Froesch, E.R. (1984) Body size parallels insulin-like growth factor I levels but not growth hormone secretory capacity. *Acta Endocrinology* 106, 448–453.

Etherton, T.D. and Bauman, D.E. (1998) Biology of somatotropin in growth and lactation of domestic animals. *Physiological Reviews* 78, 745–761.

Green, H., Morikawa, M. and Nixon, T. (1985) A dual effector theory of growth-hormone action. *Differentiation* 29, 195–198.

Hossner, K.L., McCusker, R.H. and Dodson, M.V. (1997) Insulin-like growth factors and their binding proteins in domestic animals. *Animal Science* 64, 1–15.

Isaakson, O.G.P., Jansson, J.-O. and Gause, I.A.M. (1982) Growth hormone stimulates longitudinal bone growth directly. *Science* 216, 1237–1239.

Klindt, J., Yen, J.T., Buonomo, F.C., Roberts, A.J. and Wise, T. (1998) Growth, body composition and endocrine responses to chronic administration of insulin-like growth factor I and (or) porcine growth hormone in pigs. *Journal of Animal Science* 76, 2368–2381.

LeRoith, D., Bondy, C., Yakar, S., Liu, J.L. and Butler, A. (2001) The somatomedin hypothesis: 2001. *Endocrine Reviews* 22, 53–74.

McGrane, M.M., Yun, J.S., Moorman, A.F.M., Lamers, W.H., Hendrick, G.K., Arafah, B.M., Park, E.A., Wagner, T.E. and Hanson, R.W. (1990) Metabolic effects of developmental, tissue-, and cell-specific expression of a chimeric phosphoenolpyruvate carboxykinase (Grp)/bovine growth hormone gene in transgenic mice. *Journal of Biological Chemistry* 265, 22371–22379.

Moseley, W.M., Paulissen, J.B., Goodwin, M.C., Alaniz, G.R. and Claflin, W.H. (1992) Recombinant bovine somatotropin improves growth performance in finishing beef steers. *Journal of Animal Science* 70, 412–425.

Palmiter, R.D., Brinster, R.L., Hammer, R.E., Trumbauer, M.E., Rosenfeld, M.G., Birnberg, N.C. and Evans, R.M. (1982) Dramatic growth of mice that develop from eggs microinjected with metallothionein–growth hormone fusion genes. *Nature* 300, 611–615.

Powell-Braxton, L., Hollingshead, P., Warburton, C., Dowd, M., Pitts-Meek, S., Dalton, D., Gillett N. and Stewart, T.A. (1993) IGF-I is required for normal embryonic growth in mice. *Genes and Development* 7, 2609–2617.

Salmon, W.D. and Daughaday, W.H. (1957) A hormonally controlled serum factor which stimulates sulfate incorporation by cartilage *in vitro*. *The Journal of Laboratory and Clinical Medicine* 49, 825–836.

Schlechter, N.L., Russell, S.M., Spencer, E.M. and Nicoll, C.S. (1986) Evidence suggesting that the direct growth-promoting effect of growth hormone on cartilage *in vivo* is mediated by local production of somatomedin. *Proceedings of the Natural Academy of Sciences USA* 83, 7932–7934.

Schoenle, E., Zapf, J., Humbel, R.E. and Froesch, E.R. (1982) Insulin-like growth factor I stimulates growth in hypophysectomized rats. *Nature* 296, 252–253.

Schoenle, E., Zapf, J., Hauri, C., Steiner, T. and Froesch, E.R. (1985) Comparison of *in vivo* effects of insulin-like growth factors I and II and of growth hormone in hypophysectomized rats. *Acta Endocrinology* 108, 167–174.

6 Calcium Homeostasis and Regulation of Bone Growth

Bone provides the structure for muscle attachment and locomotion and allows us to maintain our body form. Although one does not usually consider bone as a physiologically active organ, bone is an active organ system that respires, metabolizes substrates and is in a constant flux, growing and changing shape throughout an animal's lifetime. In adult humans, the entire skeleton is replaced about every 10 years. Bone is continually changing shape, especially in the growing animal. The shapes of bones are altered by removing bony matrix through the process called bone resorption and replacing the resorbed bone by synthesis and deposition of new bone. The processes of bone resorption and deposition are tightly linked and existing bone is dissolved and resorbed by osteoclasts at the same time as new bone matrix is deposited by osteoblasts. Bone also acts as a reservoir or storage site for several important minerals, especially calcium and phosphate, which are found in the circulation.

Bones contain 99% of the body's calcium and 85% of the phosphate. Calcium and phosphate play important roles in regulating homeostatic processes in animals. For example, calcium is an important cofactor in the process of blood clot formation and, along with Na^+ and K^+, helps to maintain the transmembrane potential of cells. This is essential for maintenance and regulation of nerve and muscle excitability as well as the maintenance of all cellular functions. In addition, calcium serves as a cofactor for several enzymes and, as we have seen, is essential in the activation of many intracellular messengers for the endocrine system. Phosphate is an important component in many biological molecules, including nucleotides, nucleic acids, phospholipids, proteins and enzymes. Calcium and phosphate are stored in bone as hydroxyapatite, $Ca_{10}(PO_4)_6(OH)_2$, the insoluble form of the bone mineral matrix. After deposition by osteoblasts and osteocytes, hydroxyapatite precipitates on the organic collagen matrix in alkaline environments. Hydroxyapatite is solubilized in acidic environments, in response to reduced blood Ca^{2+}. This chapter will first outline the effects of hormones on calcium homeostasis and then will examine the regulation of bone growth and differentiation by hormones and growth factors.

Hormonal Regulation of Calcium Homeostasis

Regulation and maintenance of blood calcium levels involves a balance between sources of circulating calcium and mechanisms to remove calcium from the bloodstream. Calcium in the circulation is derived from calcium ingested in the diet and absorbed by the small intestine, and from mobilization of calcium from the skeleton. Regulation of blood calcium levels occurs at the organ level in the intestinal epithelium and the kidneys. In the intestinal epithelium, calcium from the diet is actively transported into the circulation. The kidneys regulate circulating calcium concentrations through the processes of calcium excretion and reabsorption (Fig. 6.1). These processes, essential for the maintenance of calcium homeostasis, are regulated in large part by the endocrine system. The three major hormones which regulate the intestinal uptake, renal excretion and bone homeostasis of calcium and phosphate are parathyroid hormone (PTH), 1,25-dihydroxy vitamin D_3 (1,25-$(OH)_2$-D_3) and calcitonin (CT). Both PTH and vitamin D elevate blood calcium concentrations in response to lowered serum calcium, while CT reduces blood calcium in response to elevated calcium. The relationships between these hormones are shown in Fig. 6.2.

Parathyroid hormone

PTH is synthesized by the four parathyroid glands, two of which are embedded on the back of each of the paired thyroid glands. The presence of PTH is essential for life. While other hormones are needed for normal body function, they are not essential for survival. The essential nature of PTH is

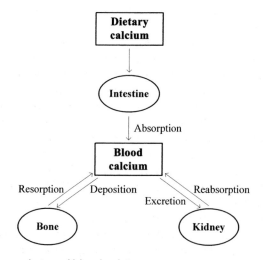

Fig. 6.1. Homeostatic regulation of blood calcium.

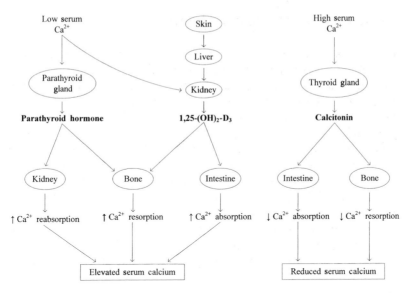

Fig. 6.2. Hormonal regulation of calcium homeostasis.

demonstrated by the consequences of removing PTH. Historically, when the thyroid glands were surgically removed, the existence of the parathyroid glands was unknown and these were unwittingly removed along with thyroids. This resulted in a rapid decline in blood calcium, followed by tetanic convulsions and death.

PTH is a single-chain polypeptide consisting of 84 amino acids. Its molecular weight is ~9600. PTH is released from the parathyroid glands in response to reduced blood calcium concentrations. The primary targets for PTH are the kidneys and osteoblast cells in the bone. The biological effects of PTH are mediated by membrane-bound G-protein-linked PTH receptors in target tissues.

Biologically, PTH has several effects on calcium homeostasis. In general, PTH induces an elevation of blood calcium, while reducing blood phosphate. It does this through three separate mechanisms. In the kidney, PTH has a direct effect, increasing tubular reabsorption of calcium while increasing phosphate excretion. PTH also has an indirect effect on the kidney, where it stimulates $1,25\text{-}(OH)_2\text{-}D_3$ synthesis. $1,25\text{-}(OH)_2\text{-}D_3$, in turn, acts on the small intestine to increase calcium absorption from the diet. In bone, PTH enhances bone resorption and the release of calcium and phosphate by effects on osteoblasts and osteoclasts. As bone resorption is the primary function of osteoclasts, it was thought that PTH effects on bone resorption were due to the direct effects of PTH on osteoclasts. Like many hormones and growth factors that stimulate bone resorption by osteoclasts, the effects of PTH are indirect, and mediated by osteoblasts. Osteoblasts, after stimulation by PTH, activate osteoclasts to undergo differentiation and initiate bone resorption. This unique relationship between osteoblasts and osteoclasts was

Table 6.1. Demonstration of the indirect effect of PTH on bone resorption.

Cells/hormone	Surface area resorbed ($\mu m^2 \times 10^{-3}$)
Osteoclasts alone	3.8
Osteoclasts + PTH	4.8
Osteoclasts + osteoblasts	2.8
Osteoclasts + osteoblasts + PTH	8.4

Source: McSheehy and Chambers (1986).

first demonstrated using an *in vitro* system to study bone resorption. In this system, isolated osteoblasts and osteoclasts, alone or in combination, are grown on slices of human femoral bone. The bone surfaces were then evaluated for the amount of bone that was degraded by measuring the surface area of the osteoclast-created pits created by osteoclasts during the incubation period (Table 6.1).

This study showed that when osteoclasts alone were treated with PTH, there was no increase in bone resorption over that of untreated osteoclasts. In addition, the co-culture of osteoblasts and osteoclasts, without hormonal stimulation, did not induce bone resorption. However, when osteoblasts and osteoclasts were grown together and stimulated with PTH, the bone resorption area was more than doubled compared to the untreated co-cultures. Thus, PTH does not act directly on osteoclasts to increase bone resorption. The induction of osteoclastic bone resorption by PTH requires the presence of osteoblasts. PTH-stimulated osteoblasts, in turn, signal osteoclasts to increase bone resorption. It is now known that this interaction between PTH, osteoblasts and osteoclasts is mediated by a unique cell-to-cell interaction system, the RANK/RANKL system, which was discussed in Chapter 4.

1,25-Dihydroxy vitamin D$_3$

1,25-Dihydroxy vitamin D$_3$, commonly known as vitamin D, is a steroid that is synthesized within the body, circulates in the bloodstream and acts via specific receptors in target cells. It is an essential regulatory factor in maintaining the homeostasis of blood and bone calcium. Vitamin D does not fulfil the classical definition of a vitamin, that is, a substance essential for normal metabolism and growth that is provided by dietary sources. Vitamin D is synthesized in the body and external sources are not normally required for adequate metabolism. However, as the precursor vitamin D was first identified as an essential nutrient, it is still classified as a fat-soluble vitamin. Vitamin D might be better described as a prohormone, as it is a precursor to the biologically active hormone, 1,25-(OH)$_2$ vitamin D$_3$.

As shown in Figs. 6.3 and 6.4, the synthesis of active 1,25-(OH)$_2$ vitamin D$_3$ is accomplished by the cooperation of multiple organs. The steroid pre-

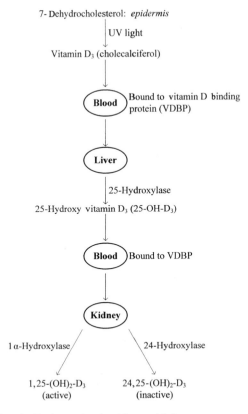

7- Dehydrocholesterol: *epidermis*

↓ UV light

Vitamin D₃ (cholecalciferol)

Blood — Bound to vitamin D binding protein (VDBP)

Liver

25-Hydroxylase

25-Hydroxy vitamin D₃ (25-OH-D₃)

Blood — Bound to VDBP

Kidney

1 α-Hydroxylase / 24-Hydroxylase

1,25-(OH)₂-D₃ (active)   24,25-(OH)₂-D₃ (inactive)

Fig. 6.3. $1,25\text{-}(OH)_2$-Vitamin D_3 is synthesized by multiple organs.

cursor, 7-dehydrocholesterol, is a cholesterol derivative that is converted in the epidermis into the prohormone vitamin D_3 (also called cholecalciferol), a reaction that is catalysed by the ultraviolet portion of sunlight. In the bloodstream cholecalciferol is bound to a protein called vitamin D-binding protein (VDBP). In the liver, cholecalciferol is hydroxylated to form 25-hydroxy vitamin D_3. This, in turn, is transported by VDBP in the circulation to the kidney, where it is further hydroxylated in the mitochondria by the enzyme 1α-hydroxylase into the active $1,25\text{-}(OH)_2\text{-}D_3$. Another enzyme in the kidney, 24-hydroxylase, can convert the 25-hydroxy vitamin D_3 precursor into an inactive metabolite, $24,25\text{-}(OH)_2\text{-}D_3$.

Biological actions of 1,25-dihydroxy vitamin D_3

$1,25$-Dihydroxy vitamin D_3, or vitamin D, acts via a nuclear steroid receptor in its target tissues. Binding of vitamin D activates the vitamin D receptor (VDR) and the receptor forms dimers with other VDR molecules. This activated receptor complex then interacts with specific enhancer and promoter sequences of specific genes in the nucleus to activate or repress their expression.

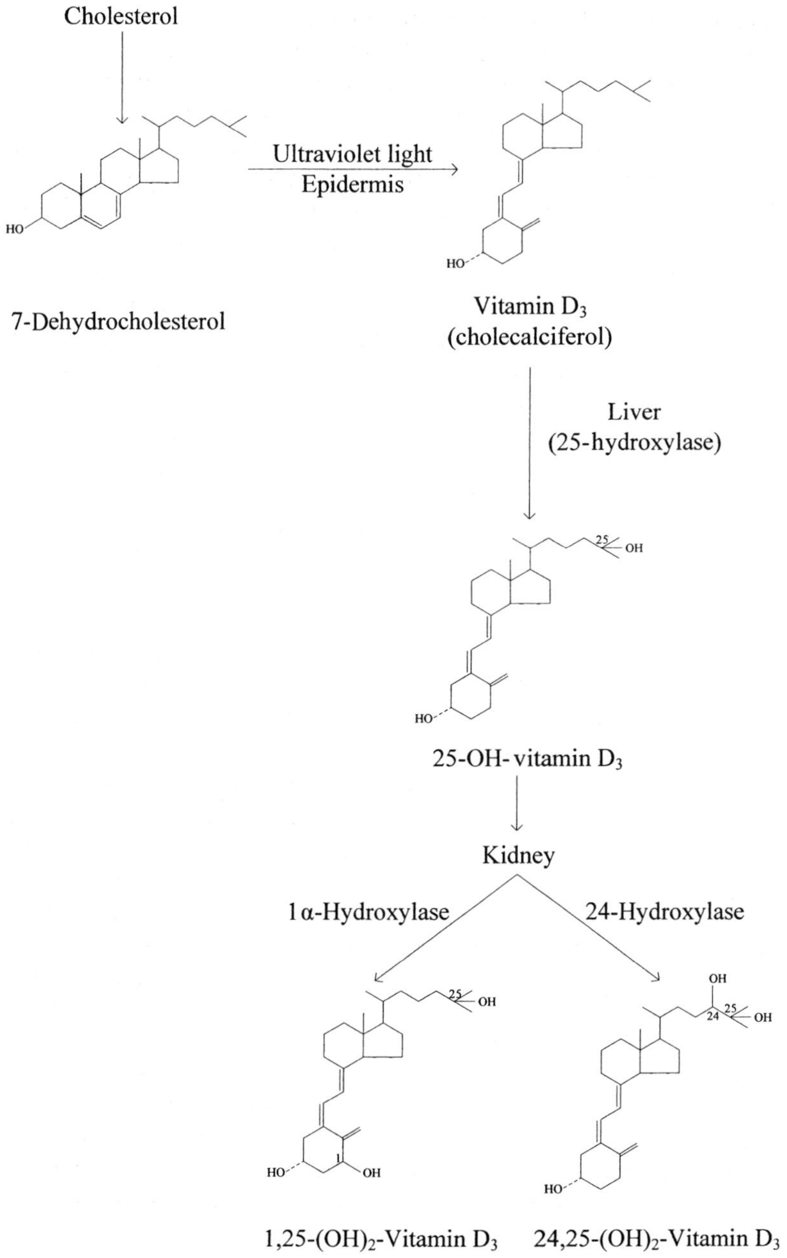

Fig. 6.4. Chemical structure and synthesis of biologically active 1,25-(OH)$_2$ vitamin D$_3$.

The main target organs affected by vitamin D are the small intestine, the kidney and bone. The primary effect of vitamin D is in the intestine, where it stimulates the uptake of dietary calcium by the intestinal epithelium. The trophic effect of vitamin D on bone mineralization may actually be a secondary or indirect effect of vitamin D. Thus, the effects on bone growth and mineralization may be due simply to the provision of adequate dietary calcium for bone formation. For example, in knockout mice lacking the VDR or in vitamin D-deficient individuals, the effects of vitamin D deficiency on bone can be overcome simply by providing supplementary calcium and phosphate in the diet.

In the intestine, vitamin D enhances calcium uptake from the diet by increasing the synthesis of an intracellular calcium transport protein called calbindin. Calbindin ferries calcium from the intestinal luminal side of the cell to the basal portion of the cell. Calcium transport out of the intestinal epithelial cell occurs against a concentration gradient, and secretion from the cell requires the active transport of calcium by a calcium pump. Vitamin D also induces the synthesis of the calcium pump mRNA and protein. Hence, vitamin D induces the uptake and delivery of dietary calcium into the bloodstream.

Vitamin D is required for bone mineralization. Animals deficient in vitamin D are characterized by the development of poorly mineralized bones. In children, this results in a syndrome called rickets, while in adults vitamin D deficiency causes a similar pathological state called osteomalacia. Both result in mineral-deficient, soft, flexible bones that are incapable of adequately supporting the body and deform under the normal stress of body support. While the effects of vitamin D on mineral homeostasis *in vivo* are well known and are centred on the stimulation of bone mineralization, vitamin D treatment of bone cells *in vitro* stimulates the formation of osteoclasts. This effect of vitamin D on osteoclast formation is indirect, mediated by the VDR in osteoblasts and the subsequent expression of RANKL in osteoblasts. Activation of the RANK/RANKL system in osteoblasts and osteoclasts stimulates the differentiation and activation of osteoclasts and results in bone resorption. As bone mineralization and remodelling is coupled to bone resorption, activation of osteoclasts by vitamin D is likely a complementary portion of the bone remodelling system, as bone synthesis is coupled to bone resorption. Vitamin D also stimulates the production of the non-collagenous matrix proteins, osteocalcin and osteonectin, in osteoblast cultures *in vitro*. Thus, in addition to its role in calcium and phosphate homeostasis, vitamin D has effects on the skeleton that are related to bone remodelling and bone turnover.

The production of vitamin D is stimulated by calcium and phosphate deficiencies. Reduction of phosphate is detected in the kidney, which increases vitamin D synthesis, while the effects of reduced calcium are mediated by an increase in PTH secretion, which stimulates vitamin D synthesis and secretion by the kidney. Elevated levels of vitamin D enhance the PTH-stimulated reabsorption of calcium by the distal tubules by increasing the synthesis of the PTH receptor in the distal tubule. Elevated calcium levels, as well as elevated vitamin D itself, directly inhibit the vitamin D 1α-hydroxylase enzyme in the kidney and reduce the synthesis of $1,25\text{-}(OH)_2\text{-}D_3$.

Calcitonin

CT is the third major hormonal player in the regulation of bone and blood calcium. The primary source of CT is the C-cells (parafollicular cells) of the thyroid gland. The major cell types of the thyroid gland are the follicular cells, which are responsible for thyroid hormone secretion. The parafollicular cells comprise a minor proportion of thyroid gland cells and are dispersed throughout the thyroid gland, but occur mainly in the central region of the gland. In addition, CT has been found in several organs in the body, including the thymus, small intestine, urinary bladder, lung and liver in humans. CT is a small polypeptide, consisting of 32 amino acids, with a molecular weight of 3410 Da. CT is a product of the CT gene family, which consists of five genes: CALC I, II, III, IV and V. CALC-I is the source of human CT. These genes also produce other family members including CT gene-related peptides I and II, adrenomedullin, amylin and other peptides present in the circulation. Members of this family are characterized by a single disulphide bond that links the amino terminal cysteine and a cysteine at position 7, forming a ring structure containing seven amino acids. The carboxy terminal end of this family of peptides is characterized by the presence of an amide cap.

The plasma membrane receptor for CT was cloned in 1991 from porcine kidney cells. The receptor belongs to the G-protein-linked receptor family. It is a seven transmembrane-domain receptor that consists of 482 amino acids. Activation of the receptor by CT binding induces several different intracellular transduction pathways, including induction of adenylate cyclase and cAMP production, and activation of PKA as well as the phosphoinositide-dependent pathway involving PLC and intracellular Ca^{2+} mobilization. Activation of a specific pathway depends not only on target cell type, but also may vary according to the stage of the cell cycle of the target cell. CT receptors are widespread throughout the body, occurring in the CNS and reproductive tissues, where their function is largely unknown. The distribution of CT receptors and CT-producing cells in the body suggests a wider role of CT in general metabolism. Of interest to the metabolism and homeostasis of calcium, CT receptors are present in the major target organs, the kidneys and the osteoclasts.

CT was initially isolated in the 1960s as a hypocalcaemic factor, on the basis of its ability to reduce serum calcium concentrations. The precise role of CT in the normal physiological regulation of calcium remains uncertain. Studies of the function of CT are flawed by the use of CT derived from unique animal species, including the salmon and eel, the use of rodents, the widespread synthesis of CT in the body and the use of pharmacological doses to elicit responses. CT is released into the bloodstream in response to Ca^{2+} infusion. When animals are treated with CT, there is an acute reduction of serum levels of calcium, but the magnitude of this response varies with animal and CT species, dose and injection route. CT reduces blood calcium levels by increasing the excretion of calcium by the kidneys and by the inhibition of bone resorption.

CT inhibits bone resorption by direct effects on osteoclasts, initially inhibiting the motility of osteoclasts, followed by the retraction of osteoclast pseudopods that contact the bone surface. Then it is followed by a CT-induced alteration of the characteristic morphology of the osteoclasts and the osteoclasts form small, rounded and non-motile cells. These morphological changes are accompanied by loss of the typical biochemical profile of the osteoclasts. The carbonic anhydrase activity and the acid phosphatase activity, characteristically elevated in active osteoclasts, are reduced by very small concentrations (picomolar) of CT. Chronic treatment with CT reduces the number of osteoclasts in bone as well as the levels of urinary hydroxyproline, an amino acid marker of bone resorption. Because of the effects of CT on reducing osteoclast activity and function, CT is used to treat bone loss and rapid bone turnover diseases. It is also used to correct hypercalcaemic disorders that result from mobilization of calcium from the skeletal system.

Regulation of Bone Growth and Development

The hedgehogs and early skeletal differentiation

Cell-to-cell signalling is a critical component of tissue and organ development in the early embryo. Only five signal transduction pathways control the early development of tissues in most animals. These cellular signals consist of wingless (Wnt), TGF-β, notch, receptor tyrosine kinase (RTK) and the hedgehogs. The hedgehogs act as paracrine agents secreted by embryonic cells that induce differentiation of specific adjacent tissues during embryonic development. These molecules are called morphogens due to their distinct effect on inducing morphological changes. The hedgehogs, notch and wingless were first discovered in the fruit fly, *Drosophila melanogaster*, and were named after the mutant fruit fly phenotypes.

The hedgehogs determine the fate of undifferentiated precursor cells, providing inductive cues to these cells and committing them into specific differentiation pathways. Embryos with the hedgehog mutation are covered with pointed denticles, resembling a hedgehog. At present, there are three known hedgehog genes in vertebrates: sonic hedgehog (SHH), Indian hedgehog (IHH) and desert hedgehog (DHH). Two of the genes are named after species of hedgehog (Indian and desert) and sonic hedgehog is named after a video game. The hedgehogs act on target cells through specific plasma membrane receptors with 12 transmembrane domains called patched (Ptc). Smoothened (Smo) is a seven transmembrane co-receptor that does not bind hedgehogs, but inhibits the constitutive activation of the Ptc signal. Binding of the hedgehog ligand to Ptc removes the constitutive inhibition of Smo and allows induction of intracellular signals and the subsequent activation of specific genes. The hedgehogs have been implicated in the differentiation and development of major portions of the body, including the brain, spinal cord, eyes, limbs and craniofacial regions as well as the skeleton. In the skeleton, SHH is expressed in the embryonic limb bud where it induces mesenchymal determination and limb formation. SHH also induces early chondrocyte differentiation and osteocyte maturation. IHH acts as a mitogen in the skeletal system, stimulating chondrocyte proliferation while slowing differentiation.

Regulation of bone growth and differentiation by hormones

Unlike the hormones discussed above, PTH, CT and vitamin D, which regulate mineral homeostasis in bone and blood, the hormones described in this section are involved with bone cell replication, differentiation, maturation and maintenance of the differentiated state. In this section, the effects of the GH/IGF system, glucocorticoids, sex steroids and thyroid hormones on bone growth and development are discussed.

The GH/IGF-I system is a primary regulatory system in bone, and is essential for the development and maintenance of the differentiated function of bone tissue. Many of the effects of the IGF/GH system are discussed in Chapter 5. Several studies have been conducted to distinguish between the effects of GH and IGF-I on bone. The complexity of the GH/IGF system makes it difficult to separate the action of these factors. GH and IGF-I act as hormones and circulating concentrations of these factors have effects on distant target tissues. In addition, the IGFs are produced locally in most, or all of the tissues in the body, where they act as growth factors without the intervention of the circulatory system. Before the mid-1980s, there was a great deal of controversy about the role of endocrine GH and IGF-I in stimulating long bone growth. This controversy was settled when Isaksson showed that the effects of GH on long bone growth were mediated by local bone production of IGF-I. It is now believed that GH stimulates bone precursor mesenchymal cells to differentiate and express IGF-I and the IGF-I receptor. IGF-I then acts in an autocrine manner to enhance clonal mitotic growth of these cells and to maintain their differentiated function. This is known as the dual effector hypothesis of GH and IGF action, as described in Chapter 5.

Recent studies have shown that IGF-I and IGF-II are found in abundance in bone and that the IGFs play critical roles in the regulation of bone growth and development. Although the IGFs are also present in the circulation at high concentrations, the local secretion and activity of IGFs in the bone are believed to be the primary mechanism by which IGFs regulate bone growth. Both IGF-I and IGF-II are present in the bone, but the activities of one form vs the other have not been adequately examined. The majority of studies have used cells derived from laboratory rodents or humans and the effects of IGF-I and IGF-II vary according to species, cell type and the stage of differentiation of the cells studied. Both IGF-I and IGF-II are synthesized and secreted by osteoblasts. They are stored in the bony ECM and their effects are modulated by the presence of IGF-binding proteins in the matrix. The actions of both forms are believed to be mediated by the Type I IGF receptor, which is present in osteoblasts and osteoclasts.

Both IGF-I and IGF-II can induce the formation of bone *in vivo* and *in vitro*. The original studies that identified the IGFs as growth factors used a cartilage system to show that factors induced by GH were responsible for cartilage and bone growth. The IGFs are generally thought of as mitogenic factors, but in bone they also play important roles in the recruitment of precursor cells to the osteoblast and osteoclast cell lineage and function in the maintenance of the differentiated state of bone. The IGFs stimulate the proliferation of pluripotent bone marrow stromal cells, thus providing an increased population of precursor cells available for differentiation into osteoblasts. IGFs do not induce differentiation of these cells, as indicated by the lack of induction of a specific transcription factor, Cbfa1, that is essential for commitment of precursor cells to the osteoblast lineage. Commitment and differentiation of these cells is regulated by other growth factors and morphogens. After differentiation into osteoblasts, the IGFs induce the synthesis of typical proteins characteristic of the differentiated state, such as Type I collagen and other matrix proteins. The IGFs also reduce collagenase expression by osteoblasts. Thus, the effects of IGFs on bone cells depend upon the state of differentiation of these cells. The IGFs act as mitogens for the undifferentiated precursor cells and maintain the differentiated function of mature osteoblasts.

The IGFs also have direct and indirect effects on osteoclasts, inducing recruitment, formation and activation of these bone-resorbing cells. The IGFs stimulate migration of precursor haematopoietic cells, the formation of the multinucleated osteoclasts and the secretion of tartrate-resistant acid phosphatase, a biochemical marker of activated osteoclasts. In mature osteoclasts, IGF-I, but not IGF-II, induces bone resorption. This effect is indirect, as osteoblasts must be present for induction of bone resorption, and may be mediated by the intercellular osteoblast–osteoclast RANK/RANKL system described in Chapter 4.

The expression of IGFs by osteoblasts varies with developmental stage and the differentiation state of these cells. As osteoblasts differentiate, the secretion of IGF-I is reduced while IGF-II secretion is increased. This has led to the suggestion that IGF-II may be the more important IGF in bone cells, but this has not been conclusively demonstrated. Circulating hormones and local growth factors also regulate the secretion of the IGFs from osteoblasts. The effects of PTH on bone growth and mineralization are mediated in part by IGF-I, as PTH treatment of osteoblasts increases IGF-I expression *in vitro* and *in vivo*. Glucocorticoids, which induce differentiation of bone marrow stromal cells into osteoblasts, suppress the synthesis of IGF-I, while increasing IGF-II expression. Other growth factors in the bone matrix also regulate the expression of the IGFs. For example bone morphogenic proteins (BMP), which induce proliferation and differentiation of osteogenic cells, induce IGF-I and IGF-II expression in osteoblasts. Potent mitogens such as fibroblast growth factor (FGF) and PDGF inhibit the expression of IGFs in osteoblasts.

The effects of glucocorticoids on bone are largely dependent upon dose. Large, pharmacological amounts of glucocorticoids are catabolic to bone formation and induce bone loss. This is seen during treatment of individuals with glucocorticoids to reduce inflammation or to suppress the immune system. Cushing's disease, characterized by the oversecretion of glucocorticoids from the adrenal gland, also induces bone loss in affected individuals. These effects may be due to indirect actions of the glucocorticoids, which reduce GH, oestrogen and testosterone secretion in the intact animal. Pharmacological doses of glucocorticoids also reduce intestinal absorption of calcium and increase calcium and phosphate excretion in the urine.

Glucocorticoids have direct effects on the kidneys, and also act indirectly, by increasing PTH and vitamin D concentrations that augment calcium excretion.

Glucocorticoids have direct effects on bone. Osteoblasts, as well as most cells in the body, have glucocorticoid receptors. Pharmacological doses (hundreds of nanomolar to micromolar range) of glucocorticoids inhibit pre-osteoblast and osteoblast DNA, RNA and protein synthesis and reduce bone formation. Proliferation and the differentiated functions of mature osteoblasts, such as collagen secretion, are inhibited by high doses of glucocorticoids. At physiological levels, in the low nanomolar range, glucocorticoids are anabolic and stimulate the differentiation of osteoblast progenitor cells and enhance bone formation. At levels comparable to those seen in the normal animal, glucocorticoids increase the differentiation of bone marrow stromal cells into the osteoblast cell lineage. At the same time, glucocorticoids inhibit the proliferation of these cells, reducing the available pool of progenitor cells and thus reducing bone formation. In differentiated osteoblasts, physiological levels of glucocorticoids maintain the differentiated state, inducing Type I collagen production, alkaline phosphatase synthesis, osteoid production and bone mineralization. Glucocorticoids also have effects on bone resorption, via the osteoclasts. Like many hormones' effects on osteoclasts, the glucocorticoids act upon osteoblasts, inducing the RANKL protein and decreasing the expression of the soluble decoy receptor, OPG, in these cells. As we have seen, this results in a stimulation of osteoclast formation and, as a result, increased bone resorption.

Many of the effects of glucocorticoids in bone, as well as other tissues, are permissive. That is, the presence of glucocorticoids is required to maintain normal cell processes, including maintenance of cell receptors for other hormones or the provision of adequate nutrients, such as glucose, for basal cell metabolism, growth and differentiation. For example, glucocorticoids induce the expression of receptors for PTH and IGF-I in osteoblasts, which allows these hormones to exert their stimulatory effects on bone. The inhibitory effects of glucocorticoids on bone formation are, in part, mediated by IGF-I, which is suppressed by glucocorticoid treatment. As the inhibitory effects of glucocorticoids persist in animals lacking IGF-I (IGF-I knockout mice), at least a portion of the effects of glucocorticoids on bone formation is due to direct actions of the glucocorticoids in bone.

As might be expected, sex steroids have definite effects on bone growth. The male hormone, testosterone, stimulates mitosis of cells in the growth plate and high testosterone levels at puberty induce closure of the growth plate. Pre-pubertal castration of males increases long bone growth due to the combined effects of testosterone deficiency and the enhanced effects of oestrogen. On the other hand, high doses of oestrogen reduce linear bone growth. In bone, oestradiol-17β stimulates OPG production of the RANK/RANKL system of osteoblasts and osteoclasts. This inhibits RANK/RANKL interactions and inhibits bone resorption by osteoclasts. When oestrogen is absent, as in ovariectomized animals or postmenopausal women, the RANK/RANKL system is active and bone resorption is increased. This results in a reduction in bone mass and bone mineralization, a condition known as osteoporosis. As with many hormones, oestrogen may also have indirect effects on bone metabolism. Treatment with oestrogen causes an increase in the circulating levels of the calcium regulatory hormones 1,25-$(OH)_2$ vitamin D_3, CT and PTH that may mediate or potentiate some of the effects of oestrogen on bone growth and mineral deposition. In non-ruminants, systemic IGF-I concentrations are reduced by oestrogen treatment, while in ruminants, there is evidence that oestrogen increases circulating concentrations of GH and IGF-I.

Thyroid hormones have direct and indirect effects on most metabolic processes in the body. They are needed to maintain metabolic rate and to modulate oxygen consumption and mitochondrial dynamics in all cells of the body. As with the glucocorticoids, many of the effects of thyroid hormones are likely to be primarily permissive in nature, providing a hormonal environment that allows the cell to metabolize energy sources and respond optimally to other hormonal stimuli. Thus, the role of thyroid hormones is largely synergistic with other hormones and growth factors that play direct roles in stimulating bone growth. In addition, thyroid hormones have distinct effects on bone growth. A lack of thyroid hormones during embryonic development leads to poor bone growth, while excess thyroid hormones cause an increase in bone resorption.

Growth factors and bone

In addition to the effects of circulating hormones, bone growth and metabolism are regulated by several polypeptide growth factors present in bone. They are synthesized and secreted by osteoblasts and other cells in bone and act in a local autocrine or paracrine manner in bone and cartilage. Upon secretion, many growth factors are bound to the ECM, which contains a variety of growth factors, including several known osteoblast mitogens and differentiation-inducing factors. The growth factors in the ECM provide a reservoir of regulatory factors, which act as autocrine and paracrine agents to direct the growth and remodelling of bone. Growth factors are not restricted to bone but are widely distributed throughout the body and are present in most, if not all, tissues. In addition, the effects of growth factors on bone growth are not tissue-specific. That is, specific growth factors are mitogens not only in bone, but also in all tissues in which they are present. In general, the synthesis and secretion of growth factors are not affected by circulating hormones. Examples of these local tissue growth factors include: FGF, PDGF, TGF, BMP as well as IGF-I and IGF-II. We will consider each of these growth factors individually in some detail.

FGF

The FGFs are also called heparin-binding growth factors and were first isolated based on their binding to heparin using immobilized heparin affinity columns. The first FGFs isolated were called acidic FGF and basic FGF (aFGF and bFGF). These forms correspond to what are now called FGF-1 and FGF-2, respectively. Since the initial isolation of FGF, it has been shown that these growth factors are part of a superfamily of polypeptides consisting of at least 23 major isoforms. These growth factors do more than simply stimulate fibroblast mitosis. The FGFs play significant roles in embryonic development and differentiation, where they induce cell migration via chemotaxis, and stimulate differentiation of the skeleton, skeletal muscle, neural tissue, blood and blood vessels. The FGF superfamily of growth factors stimulates the proliferation of a wide range of mesodermally derived and epithelial cells, including skin keratinocytes, endothelial cells, myoblasts, osteoblasts and chondrocytes.

The molecular weights of the FGF superfamily members range from 17 to 38 kDa, consisting of 160 to 288 amino acids. In general, the genes for the FGF superfamily consist of three exons. Many of the FGF family members are secreted into the extracellular space, but FGFs do not appear in the circulation. The FGFs generally exist as monomers, although dimeric forms of some FGFs are believed to be secreted. Some FGF family members are glycosylated and many are bound to heparin and heparin sulphate in the ECM. The ECM-bound FGF provides a local reservoir of mitogen that acts on adjacent or source cells via autocrine or paracrine mechanisms. FGFs act through four known cell surface-bound TK receptors.

FGFs are potent mitogens and are active in picogram levels. They stimulate mitosis of a wide range of cells, such as stem cells, bone and cartilage. In skeletal tissue, FGFs play an important role in recruitment, proliferation and differentiation of cartilage and bone cells. During bone development the FGFs are involved in the commitment of undifferentiated precursor cells into the osteogenic pathway, stimulate the proliferation of preosteoblasts and induce the differentiation of preosteoblasts into osteoblasts and finally, osteocytes. FGF-3, -4, and -5 are expressed early in embryonic development and in conjunction with TGF-β and BMP are responsible for early induction of mesoderm. FGF-8 and -10 are expressed in the early embryonic limbs and limb bud primordia and are involved in early limb development. FGF-2 and -4 are also involved in limb bud development. FGF-1 and -2 are expressed later in undifferentiated mesenchymal cells and in osteoblasts and chondroblasts. The cartilage cells of the resting and proliferating zones of the epiphyseal plate express FGF-2.

Both FGF-1 and -2 are important in bone formation and *in vitro* studies show that these FGFs control osteoblast proliferation and differentiation, acting at early and late stages of osteoblast differentiation. FGF-2 is more potent as a mitogen for osteoblasts than FGF-1. The effects of the FGFs depend upon the stage of development and the duration of exposure to FGF. While FGF-1 and -2 act as mitogens in early osteoblast development, later on FGF-2 inhibits functions associated with the differentiated state of bone, such as the inhibition of the synthesis and secretion of Type I collagen, osteocalcin and alkaline phosphatase activity. In contrast, FGF-2 stimulates the expression of the matrix protein, osteopontin.

The FGFs play crucial roles in postnatal bone growth and remodelling in the intact animal. Treatment of growing postnatal laboratory animals with FGF-2 stimulates bone formation and increased mineral density. The loss of bone formation and volume that results from lack of oestrogen in ovariectomized animals is restored by treatment with FGF-1 and FGF-2, suggesting that the FGFs may mediate the effects of oestrogens on bone. This effect of FGF is believed to be due to recruitment and commitment of undifferentiated mesenchymal stem cells into the bone cell differentiation pathway. An important phase of bone growth is the requisite bone resorption that occurs concurrently with bone deposition. Both FGF-1 and FGF-2 increase bone resorption *in vitro*, acting via direct and indirect pathways. The FGFs induce collagenase synthesis and secretion in bone cells. FGF-2 also induces expression of the tissue inhibitors of metalloproteinases (TIMPs), which inhibit collagenase activity. Thus, the FGFs have specific distinct anabolic effects on bone formation in postnatal animals.

While many FGF effects are mediated directly, by interaction with their cell surface receptors, some of the effects of FGFs are indirect and are likely mediated by other locally produced bone matrix growth factors. Both FGF-1 and -2 induce TGF-β production in bone cells, *in vivo* and *in vitro*. TGF-β, in turn, induces the expression of FGF-2 in osteoblasts, amplifying the effects of both growth factors. FGF-2 reduces the expression of IGF-I, IGF-II and the IGF-binding proteins while increasing expression of hepatocyte growth factor (HGF) in osteoblasts.

The effects of FGF-2 on osteoblast differentiation occur in concert with other growth factors. For example, the effects of BMP-2 and FGF-2 are synergistic, and pre-treatment of osteoblasts with FGF-2 enhances the cell response to BMP-2, suggesting that FGF-2 may increase BMP receptor numbers or BMP receptor sensitivity. The expression of FGF-2 in osteoblasts is, in turn, regulated by a variety of hormones and growth factors. PTH, prostaglandins and TGF-β are all positive inducers of FGF-2 expression in osteoblasts. In addition, FGF-2 is autoinductive, inducing an increased expression of its own gene in osteoblasts.

PDGF

PDGF was originally isolated from human blood platelets and was characterized by its ability to induce mitosis in a variety of cell lines, including fibroblasts and vascular smooth muscle cells. It is now known that PDGF is present in many different organs of the body and acts as a potent mitogen and as a chemotactic agent during development and tissue repair. PDGF has a molecular weight of 28–35 kDa and consists of a disulphide-linked dimer of two dissimilar chains. The active form of PDGF is derived from two separate genes that code for an A chain and a B chain. The monomers can be combined in all combinations to produce three active PDGF dimer isoforms: AA, AB and BB. PDGF-BB is the most potent isomer in bone.

The receptors for PDGF are present as monomers in the plasma membrane. Upon activation by PDGF binding the receptors form homo- and heterodimers consisting of α and β subunits: αα, αβ and ββ. The PDGF receptors have intrinsic intracellular TK activity and, after autophosphorylation, activate PKC, PKA or induce changes in intracellular calcium. Intracellular messenger pathways are specific to cell type. The αPDGF receptor binds all PDGF isoforms with equal affinity and the βPDGF receptor binds PDGF-BB with about tenfold higher affinity than PDGF-AB. It does not bind PDGF-AA. Both PDGFα and PDGFβ receptor concentrations are upregulated by PDGF-BB.

PDGF is essential for normal embryonic development and the PDGFs and their receptors are present throughout embryonic development. In the early embryo, both A and B genes are expressed in epithelial tissues overlying mesenchymal tissue that expresses the α and β PDGF receptor genes. This provides a local paracrine system that induces mitosis and migration of mesenchymal cells. Later during embryonic development, the PDGF-A gene is expressed by the surface ectoderm overlying limb buds. Both α and β receptors are present in the limb bud mesenchyme and the perichondrium of developing long bones. In the human embryo, PDGF and its receptors are widespread, found in the placenta, blood vessels, smooth muscle and mesenchyme and throughout the CNS.

The PDGFs are not required to induce the bone phenotype *per se*, but likely to play a permissive role in the embryonic development of bone. Mutations in the PDGF-B gene or the βPDGF receptor have no specific effects on fetal skeletal system development. Deletion of the PDGF-B gene or the β receptor gene results in embryonic lethality. Embryos die during the latter part of gestation (days 17–19 in mice) due to extensive vascular haemorrhage and lack of respiratory function. More specifically, embryonic death is due to failure of the diaphragm and kidneys to develop and to the disorganized development of the capillary system. The βPDGF receptor plays an important role in the development of all muscle cells including vascular, intestinal and cardiac smooth muscle and skeletal muscle. Disruption of the PDGF-A gene results in the death of about 50% of embryos before embryonic day 10 in the mouse. Survivors live for a few weeks postpartum and are severely growth-retarded. These studies demonstrate the importance of PDGF-A and -B during normal embryonic development.

In the adult, PDGF is widely expressed in tissues derived from mesoderm, including a variety of blood cells, endothelial smooth muscle, osteoblasts, the vascular system, neurones, fibroblasts and the kidneys. Reproductive system tissues such as the mammary gland, uterus and placenta also produce PDGF. Although produced locally in many tissues, PDGF acts primarily as a systemic growth factor. The blood platelets contain large quantities of PDGF and are the primary source of circulating PDGF. PDGF is released into the bloodstream by the platelets in response to mechanical injury. In the circulation, PDGF induces responses to tissue injury including inflammation, wound healing and angiogenesis.

In the skeletal system, PDGF is involved in the regulation of osteogenesis and bone repair. As with many cells, PDGF is a potent mitogen for many cell types in bone. Osteoblasts not only produce PDGF, but also they respond to it in an autocrine manner. The mitogenic effects of PDGF are primarily on osteoblast precursor cells such as bone marrow stromal cells, fibroblasts and preosteoblasts. Mature osteoblasts are less responsive to the mitogenic effects of PDGF. Treatment with PDGF results in an increase in the populations of progenitor cells which provides a pool of precursor cells that can differentiate into osteoblasts, a process that is not regulated by PDGF. The mitogenic effects on bone precursor cells and the resulting increased progenitor cell population suggest that the primary role of PDGF in the skeletal system is in the regulation of bone repair and osteogenesis.

PDGF has pronounced effects on bone remodelling and especially bone resorption, acting on both osteoclasts and osteoblasts. PDGF treatment increases the number and bone-resorbing activity of osteoclasts. Exposure of osteoblasts *in vitro* to PDGF inhibits the differentiated functions of these cells. This is reflected by the reduced alkaline phosphatase activity and the reduced secretion of Type I collagen. In addition, PDGF reduces osteoblast expression of specific bone ECM components such as osteocalcin and osteonectin. As osteonectin binds and inactivates PDGF-B in the ECM, reduction in osteonectin concentrations by PDGF may enhance the biological activity of PDGF in bone. In addition, PDGF increases the osteoblast secretion of collagenase and gelatinase, enzymes that are involved in the degradation of the organic matrix, or osteoid, of bone. PDGF induces the expression of collagenases 1 and 3 in fibroblasts and osteoblasts, respectively, and reduces collagen matrix secretion in rat calvariae. Thus, PDGF is closely associated with organic matrix degradation, a process essential in bone resorption, remodelling and turnover.

The effects of PDGF on bone may be modulated by other growth factors. Hormones that are active in bone such as PTH, 1,25-$(OH)_2$-D_3, cortisol and IGF-I have no effect on the activity or binding of PDGF to osteoblasts. In contrast, growth factors such as the interleukins, TNF-α and TGF-β regulate PDGF binding and activity in bone. Interleukins, cytokines that are primarily involved in the regulation of the growth and differentiation of blood cells, enhance osteoblast sensitivity to PDGF by increasing expression of the αPDGF receptor, enhancing the mitogenic effect of PDGF-AA. TNF-α also increases PDGF binding to the αPDGF receptors. TGF-β1, on the other hand, reduces binding of PDGF-AA and its mitogenic effects in rat and human osteoblasts.

Effects of PDGFs on bone are also indirect, mediated by other growth factors present in the skeleton. While the IGFs are present in large concentrations in the bone, their effects largely oppose those of PDGFs. For example, the IGFs induce Type I collagen synthesis and secretion while reducing collagenase expression, both functions related to the maintenance of the differentiated state of osteoblasts. Treatment of osteoblasts with PDGF reduces IGF-I and IGF-II mRNA in these cells. In osteoblasts, PDGF-BB also reduces the expression of IGFBP-5, a binding protein that potentiates the anabolic actions of IGF in bone. These effects on the reduction of IGF activity in osteoblasts enhance the effects of PDGF on collagen degradation and organic matrix turnover.

In the intact animal, treatment with PDGF-BB prevents bone loss and maintains spinal bone density in oestrogen-deficient ovariectomized rats. This occurs due to an increase in osteoblast numbers with a resultant increase in bone formation without effects on osteoclast cell numbers. As emphasized above, osteoblast cell numbers are increased due to the effects of PDGF on the replication of preosteoblasts and other stem cells. In the adult animal, PDGF-AA gene expression is increased locally in many cell types in the region of bone fractures. PDGF-BB expression is increased primarily in the osteoblasts in the area of the fracture. As PDGF is also released in large quantities by aggregating platelets in response to bone fracture and the accompanying tissue damage, systemic as well as locally produced PDGF is believed to contribute to bone fracture (and wound) healing.

Transforming growth factor-β

The TGFs were originally isolated based on their effects on cell transformation. When normal cells are grown *in vitro*, their growth is limited by contact inhibition. This means that when these cells contact another cell, they stop growing. In contrast, transformed cells, such as those that have assumed a cancerous phenotype, continue to grow when in contact with other cells. These cells will eventually overgrow one another, forming thick, flattened stacks of cells, similar to the uncontrolled neoplastic growth of cancer cells seen *in vivo*. In addition, normal cells cannot grow when suspended in agar. The TGFs were initially characterized by their ability to stimulate DNA synthesis, induce loss of contact inhibition and anchorage-independent cell colony formation of cells grown in agar. Thus, the TGFs induce a state similar to that of a transformed, tumourigenic cell. The TGFs are involved in the development of specific diseases involved with overproduction of ECM, autoimmune diseases and carcinogenesis. The focus of this section is on the effects of the TGFs on normal tissue development and differentiation. The TGFs are both mitogens and inducers of differentiation in normal cells, acting via autocrine, paracrine and endocrine modes.

There are two major divisions of the TGF family: TGF-α and TGF-β. TGF-α was first isolated from the transformed 3T3 fibroblast cell line. TGF-α is a 5600 Da polypeptide that shares a 40% amino acid sequence identity with EGF. TGF-α is considered to be an EGF-like molecule. TGF-α binds to the EGF receptor and has mitogenic activity, similar to EGF. The focus of this section will be on TGF-β.

The TGF-β superfamily consists of over 50 different molecules derived from a common ancestral gene. In addition to TGF-β, this family includes bone morphogenetic proteins, the activins, inhibins and Mullerian-inhibiting substance. The TGF-β molecules are dimers that consist of two polypeptide chains covalently linked with disulphide bonds. Three molecular isoforms, TGF-β1, -2 and -3, are produced by three separate genes. TGF-β1 is the most abundant of the isoforms. Although heterodimers of TGF-β exist, the isoforms are usually homodimers. TGF-β is secreted by cells as a large, inactive precursor molecule (~100 to 220 kDa), which is bound to the ECM. The large precursor molecule is cleaved in the ECM by proteases such as plasmin to form the active TGF-β molecule (24 kDa) and a TGF-β-binding protein. Local acidic environments, such as those induced by osteoclasts during bone resorption, also activate TGF-β and allow it to be involved in the bone remodelling process.

All isoforms of TGF-β bind to the same dimeric receptor complex that consists of two receptor types. Binding of TGF-β ligands to the Type II TGF-β receptor (75–85 kDa) induces association of this molecule with the 50–60 kDa Type I receptor, forming an activated heteromeric receptor complex that consists of Type II and Type I polypeptides. The TGF-β receptor is a serine/threonine kinase. It catalyses the phosphorylation of serine and threonine residues in the receptor itself and in downstream cytoplasmic messenger molecules.

The cytoplasmic mediators of the TGF-β family of receptors are called Smads, messenger molecules present in organisms from worms and fruit flies to mammals. There are nine vertebrate Smads resulting from three types of Smad genes: receptor-activated, common and inhibitory. Receptor-activated Smads are phosphorylated by the receptor kinase in response to ligand binding. Smads 2 and 3 are the major receptor-activated messengers for activin and TGF-β, respectively. Smads 1, 5 and 8 mediate BMP receptor actions. After they are phosphorylated by the TGF-β receptor, the receptor-activated Smads associate with the common Smad (Smad4) in the cytoplasm, forming a heterodimer that is translocated to the nucleus where it alters the transcriptional activity of specific genes. The third type of Smad, the inhibitory or anti-Smads, inhibits signalling by the receptor-activated and common Smad complex. Smad6 and Smad7 are inhibitory Smads for TGF-β, activin and BMP signalling. Unlike conventional transcription factors that bind directly to promoter sequences in genes, the Smad molecules bind to other transcription factors that are already bound to specific gene promoter sites. Interaction of Smads with other transcription factors at the gene level provides a cooperative modulation of specific gene expression.

Most cells express TGF-β and have receptors for TGF-β, indicating the importance of the autocrine function of TGF-β. In addition, TGF-β induces the expression of its own gene, prolonging TGF-β secretion and enhancing its autocrine effects. There are large quantities of TGF-β in platelets and bone tissue where they regulate normal physiological processes. Unlike many growth factors, low levels of TGF-β1 are always present in the circulation, although the definitive site of production of this endocrine TGF-β1 is unknown. Plasma levels of TGF-β1 are elevated in response to injury when it is released from platelets involved in clot formation. TGF-β2 and TGF-β3 are not present in plasma and act at local sites within tissues as autocrine and paracrine regulators of metabolism.

TGF-β inhibits the growth of most epithelial, endothelial and haematopoietic cell lineages. The inhibitory effects of TGF-β on cell growth are antagonistic to those of typical mitogenic growth factors such as FGF and PDGF. TGF-β has many effects on the ECM of bone, a function that is related to tissue repair and remodelling. TGF-β increases the expression of ECM proteins, such as fibronectin, collagen and decorin, while suppressing the secretion of enzymes involved in matrix degradation, such as collagenase and elastase.

In the skeletal system TGF-β isoforms act as growth and differentiation factors (GDF) that regulate tissue differentiation and morphogenesis, bone resorption and bone fracture repair. TGF-β is found in abundance in bone and is produced and secreted by osteoblasts and chondrocytes, which also respond to TGF-β in an autocrine manner. TGF-β and the Type I and Type II TGF-β receptors are expressed during the early embryonic differentiation of both endochondral and intramembranous bone. TGF-β is an important molecular signal that induces the differentiation of mesenchymal cells into chondrocytes and osteoblasts. Low levels of the three TGF-β isoforms are expressed in mesenchymal cells, and expression of the isoforms by these cells increases as mesenchymal cells form condensations in the areas of future endochondral bone formation. The same increased expression of TGF-β is seen in intramembranous bone mesenchymal cells that will differentiate into the osteoblasts.

In general, the physiological role of TGF-β in bone is to expand the progenitor cell population, increasing the pool of potential osteoblasts. TGF-β is mitogenic for fibroblasts, undifferentiated mesenchymal cells, osteoblast progenitors and osteoblasts. The mitogenic effects of TGF-β are similar to those of PDGF, in that the predominant TGF-β effects are to increase the number of bone precursor cells. Other growth factors and hormones regulate differentiation of this expanded population of progenitor cells into mature osteoblasts and osteocytes. Osteoblasts secrete TGF-β1 and TGF-β2 into the bone matrix, where concentration of TGF-β1 is about eightfold higher than TGF-β2. Transgenic mice that overexpress TGF-β2 in preosteoblasts have an increased number of preosteoblasts, osteoblasts and osteocytes. They are also characterized by increased bone turnover, both deposition and resorption. Although TGF-β can induce differentiation of bone marrow stromal cells into osteoblasts, the inhibitory effects of TGF-β on differentiation predominate. The stimulatory effects of PTH and vitamin D_3 on osteoblast differentiation are inhibited by TGF-β. This is reflected by the TGF-β inhibition of the expression of osteoblast alkaline phosphatase and osteocalcin in response to these hormones.

TGF-β is also produced by and has effects on the osteoclasts of the skeletal system, regulating the differentiation, activation and function of these bone-resorbing cells. Although there are conflicting views about whether TGF-β stimulates or inhibits osteoclast differentiation and bone resorption, this is likely due to dose-dependent effects. Low doses of TGF-β (picogram level), which are likely to be seen in physiological situations, stimulate osteoclast differentiation and bone resorption, while higher doses (nanogram range), which are not likely to be seen in the normal animal, inhibit osteo-clast formation. During bone resorption, the acid and proteolytic enzymes secreted by osteoclasts cleave and activate the large latent forms of TGF-β in the ECM. Active TGF-β is then able to stimulate osteoclast differentiation by at least two mechanisms that involve osteoblasts. Firstly, TGF-β stimulates osteoblasts to secrete CSF-I. CSF-I is a growth factor that is believed to stimu-late the proliferation and differentiation of osteoclast stem cells into osteo-clasts. In addition, TGF-β stimulates osteoblasts to activate the RANK/RANKL system (Chapter 4) that activates osteoclasts through their cell-to-cell contacts with osteoblasts. This results in a stimulation of osteo-clast differentiation and activation.

Bone morphogenetic proteins

The BMP are members of the TGF-β superfamily, discussed above. Historically, the BMPs have been known by a variety of names, including osteogenic protein (OP), cartilage-derived morphogenetic protein (CDMP) and GDF. This array of terminology indicates the biological effects of BMP in bone, cartilage and extraskeletal tissues. The current nomenclature of BMP is perhaps misleading, as this family of peptides has many effects outside the skeletal system. It is now known that BMPs induce a variety of cell func-tions, including stimulation of proliferation, differentiation, morphogenesis and organogenesis of many systems. Their roles are not restricted to bone development, and the BMPs might be more appropriately termed general GDFs. The activity associated with BMPs in the skeletal system was first dis-covered in the 1960s by showing that extracts of demineralized bone could induce bone formation *de novo* when implanted in ectopic sites, such as mus-cle, in rats. Ectopic treatment of non-skeletal tissues with BMP induces all of the stages of embryonic bone formation, including the initial colonization with undifferentiated mesenchymal cells that differentiate into chondrocytes, followed by osteoblast and osteoclast differentiation and bone formation.

The BMPs were first cloned and characterized biochemically in the 1980s. The BMPs share several structural features with other TGF-β family members. The BMPs are dimeric molecules, with two polypeptide chains bound covalently with disulphide bonds. Like TGF-β, the BMPs are secreted as large precursor proteins that must be proteolytically cleaved before they become biologically active. The BMP family of peptide factors now encom-passes at least 15 different members, a large proportion of the known TGF-β superfamily.

The receptor system and cytoplasmic signalling pathways for the BMPs are essentially identical to that of the TGF-βs, discussed above. The trans-membrane BMP receptors are serine/threonine kinases that are activated upon ligand binding, form dimers consisting of Type I and Type II receptors, and undergo autophosphorylation. The Type I BMP receptor subunit cataly-ses the phosphorylation of the cytoplasmic signalling molecules, the Smads. Smads 1, 5 and 8 are the receptor-activated molecules that form heteromers with the common Smad, Smad4, and mediate the signal transduction pathways of the BMPs. Smads 6 and 7 are anti-Smads that inhibit BMP, TGF-β and activin signalling.

The BMPs are expressed early in embryonic development and can be detected in day 6.5 mouse embryos; at a time that gastrulation (formation of the three germ layers) is occurring. They are widely expressed and appear in the extraembryonic membranes, such as the amnion, chorion and allantois, of the developing fetus. They are also expressed in the cardiovascular system, specifically the myocardium, mesenchymal condensations of ribs, vertebrae and in the eye and tooth primordia. Later in development they appear in chondrocytes of long bone and digits. The expression of the various isoforms of the BMPs is widespread and changes with developmental stage and tissue type. Their expression is often localized in areas of epithelial–mesenchymal tissue interactions, leading to the idea that BMPs may be involved in signalling between these embryonic tissues types.

In the adult, BMPs are believed to be involved in bone remodelling and resorption. Bones are in a continuous state of turnover or remodelling in the adult. This bone turnover involves osteoblasts and osteoclasts that respond to systemic, local and mechanical signals. The BMPs are present in the bone matrix and released at the sites of fracture. They are synthesized and secreted by osteoblasts *in vivo* and *in vitro*. Upon release, the BMPs are thought to induce mesenchymal stem cell commitment into the pre-osteoblast/osteoblast lineage. As mature osteoblasts secrete BMP, the initial induction of increased osteoblast cell numbers by BMP acts as a positive feedback pathway for BMP production, increasing BMP secretion from the enhanced populations of osteoblasts. During bone fracture repair, BMP is released at the site of fracture. All bone cells involved in fracture repair have BMP receptors and respond to BMP. Specifically, BMP2 and BMP4 released from the matrix or osteoblasts act on cells in the vicinity or recruits progenitor cells from the bone marrow to the fracture site where they differentiate into osteoblasts that modulate new bone formation and fracture repair.

References and Further Reading

Alliston, T.N. and Derynck, R. (2000) Transforming growth factor-β in skeletal development and maintenance. In: Canalis, E. (ed.) *Skeletal Growth Factors.* Lippincott, Williams & Wilkins, Philadelphia, Pennsylvania, pp. 233–249.

Conover, C.A. (2000) Insulin-like growth factors and the skeleton. In: Canalis, E., (ed.) *Skeletal Growth Factors.* Lippincott, Williams & Wilkins, Philadelphia, Pennsylvania, pp. 101–116.

Derynck, R., Zhang, Y. and Feng, X.H. (1998) Smads: transcriptional activators of TGF-beta responses. *Cell* 95, 737–740.

Gilboa, L., Nohe, A., Geissendörfer, T., Sebald, W., Henis, Y.I. and Knaus, P. (2000) Bone morphogenetic protein receptor complexes on the surface of live cells: a new oligomerization mode for serine/threonine kinase receptors. *Molecular Biology of the Cell* 11, 1023–1035.

Givol, D. and Yayon, A. (1992) Complexity of FGF receptors: genetic basis for structural diversity and functional specificity. *FASEB Journal* 6, 3362–3369.

Globus, R.K., Patterson-Buckendahl, P. and Gospodarowicz, D. (1988) Regulation of bovine bone cell proliferation by fibroblast growth factor and transforming growth factor. *Endocrinology* 123, 98–105.

Globus, R.K., Plouet, J. and Gospodarowicz, D. (1989) Cultured bovine bone cells synthesize basic fibroblast growth factor and store it in their extracellular matrix. *Endocrinology* 124, 1539–1547.

Hadley, M.E. (1984) Hormonal control of calcium homeostasis. In: Hadley, M.E. (ed.) *Endocrinology*. Prentice-Hall, Englewood Cliffs, New Jersey, pp. 182–207.

Heldin, C.-H. and Westermark, B. (1989) Platelet-derived growth factors: a family of isoforms that bind to two distinct receptors. *British Medical Bulletin* 45, 453–464.

Hock, J.M. and Canalis, E. (1994) Platelet-derived growth factor enhances bone cell replication, but not differentiated function of osteoblasts. *Endocrinology* 134, 1423–1428.

Hogan, B.L. (1996) Bone morphogenetic proteins: multifunctional regulators of vertebrate development. *Genes and Development* 10, 1580–1594.

Hurley, M.M., Marie, P.J. and Florkiewicz, R.Z. (2002) Fibroblast growth factor (FGF) and FGF receptor families in bone. In: Bilezikian, J.P., Raisz, L.G. and Rodan, G.A. (eds) *Principles of Bone Biology*, 2nd edn. Academic Press, New York, pp. 825–851.

Kawabata, M. and Miyazono, K. (2000) Bone morphogenetic proteins. In: Canalis, E. (ed.) *Skeletal Growth Factors*. Lippincott, Williams & Wilkins, Philadelphia, Pennsylvania, pp. 269–290.

Kingsley, D.M. (1994) The TGF-beta superfamily: new members, new receptors, and new genetic tests of function in different organisms. *Genes and Development* 8, 133–146.

Marks, S.C. and Odgren, P.R. (2002) Structure and development of the skeleton. In: Bilezikian, J.P., Raisz, L.G. and Rodan, G.A. (eds) *Principles of Bone Biology*, 2nd edn. Academic Press, New York, pp. 3–15.

Marks, S.C. and Popoff, S.N. (1988) Bone cell biology: the regulation of development, structure, and function in the skeleton. *American Journal of Anatomy* 183, 1–44.

Massague, J. (1998) TGFβ signal transduction. *Annual Reviews of Biochemistry* 67, 753–791.

McSheehy, P.M. and Chambers, T.J. (1986) Osteoblastic cells mediate osteoclastic responsiveness to parathyroid hormone. *Endocrinology* 118, 824–828.

Mohan, S. and Baylink, D.J. (1996) Insulin-like growth factor system components and the coupling of bone formation to resorption. *Hormone Research* 45 (Suppl. 1), 59–62.

Nilsson, A., Ohlsson, C. Isaksson, O.G., Lindahl, A. and Isgaard, J. (1994) Hormonal regulation of longitudinal bone growth. *European Journal of Clinical Nutrition* 48, S150–S158.

Pimentel, E. (1994) *Handbook of Growth Factors*, Vol. II (Peptide Growth Factors). CRC Press, Boca Raton, Florida, 362 pp.

Reddi, A.H. (1997) Bone morphogenetic proteins: an unconventional approach to isolation of first mammalian morphogens. *Cytokine and Growth Factor Reviews* 8, 11–20.

Sakou, T. (1998) Bone morphogenetic proteins: from basic studies to clinical approaches. *Bone* 22, 591–603.

Turner, C.D. and Bagnara, J.T. (1976) Parathyroid and ultimobranchial glands: PTH, calcitonin and the cholecalciferols. In: *General Endocrinology*. W.B. Saunders, Philadelphia, Pennsylvania, pp. 225–257.

Westermark, B. and Heldin, C.-H. (1993) Platelet-derived growth factors. Structure, function and implications in normal and malignant cell growth. *Acta Oncologica* 32, 101–105.

7 Hormones, Growth Factors and Skeletal Muscle

Regulation of skeletal muscle growth and differentiation involves a plethora of factors, including intrinsic genetic controls and extracellular signals, such as morphogens, growth factors and hormones, that stimulate the developing cells via receptors and nuclear transcription factors. The outline of myogenesis and the cells involved in myogenesis were described in Chapter 4. The purpose of the current chapter is to examine the molecular mechanisms that drive the processes of skeletal muscle growth, differentiation and function.

The size and numbers of myofibres are directly related to muscle mass in the postnatal animal. During myogenesis, myoblasts proliferate, differentiate and fuse to form multinucleated myotubes and mature myofibres. Cellular proliferation and differentiation during myogenesis are separate and exclusionary events. After proliferation, myoblasts withdraw from the cell cycle and fuse with one another to form myofibres that are no longer capable of mitosis. In mammals, the numbers of myofibres are determined during the latter part of gestation, during the last 10% to 20% of gestation in cattle and pigs. The size of the myofibres is determined by a number of factors, including genetics, nutrition, exercise and the endocrine environment.

Experimental Systems to Study Myogenesis

The molecular signals that induce the myogenic pathway during embryogenesis have been discovered only within the last few years, owing to the development of extremely sensitive molecular biological tools. Much of the information on embryonic development and its regulation at the molecular level has been produced using experimental models such as the round worm, *Caenorhabditis elegans*, and the fruit fly, *Drosophila melanogaster*. The use of these small, relatively simple invertebrates with short lifespans (2 to 3 weeks) and well-characterized genetics and developmental processes have led to fundamental discoveries of the molecular mechanisms involved in development of organ systems that hold true for almost all animals. Findings from these animals have been corroborated in vertebrate species such as the chicken and mouse embryo. These animals are used because of their abundance, low cost and short embryonic and adult lifespan. Many of the proteins that act as intercellular signals and intracellular transcription factors are essentially identical in species that range from round worms to humans. This conservation of the structure and function of gene products from widely disparate organisms points to the essential nature of these biochemical signals and their central role in developmental processes that determine the form and function of the mature organism.

As we have seen, the formation of skeletal muscle in birds and mammals begins near the embryonic neural tube with the formation of pluripotent somites. These paired structures, aligned along the presumptive backbone of the embryo (embryonic neural tube), give rise to the dermis of the skin, the axial skeleton (ribs, vertebrae) and most of the animal's skeletal muscle, including the body, back and limb musculature. Formation of skeletal muscle in the limbs involves the delamination of muscle progenitor cells from the somite followed by their migration to the limb bud. In the limb bud, the progenitor cells undergo proliferation to increase precursor cell numbers and then fuse to form the mature multinucleated muscle fibres. Each of these events is strictly controlled by intrinsic genetic mechanisms and external signals.

Myogenic cell systems

In addition to studies using intact embryos to examine early muscle development, many of the effects of growth factors and hormones on skeletal muscle cell growth and differentiation are studied using isolated cells *in vitro*. Use of these cells eliminates the effects of multiple complex interactions between hormones, growth factors and nutrients that occur in the intact animal. Cells are grown in a buffered culture medium containing glucose, vitamins and minerals in an appropriate osmotic balance. Temperature, pH, oxygen and carbon dioxide are also maintained at constant levels. This allows one to study the effect of external factors in a controlled environment. Culture medium is often supplemented with serum, which is added to maintain cell survival and induce mitosis. Unfortunately, serum contains variable and unknown quantities of hormones, growth factors, vitamins and minerals. These unknowns contribute to the variation of data produced from this system. On the other hand, cells can be grown in a serum-free, defined culture medium that provides known amounts of nutrients and growth factors. Various combinations of albumin (as a protein and osmotic source), insulin, the iron-binding protein transferrin, glucocorticoids and thyroid hormones may be added in order to maintain normal cell metabolism and substitute for the lack of serum in defined media.

The use of cells maintained in an artificial environment *in vitro* to study physiological processes suffers from some drawbacks. Most obviously, cells grown in a single layer on a flat Petri dish lack the normal architecture seen in the animal. The three-dimensional relationship of the cells in the original tissue and the interaction of myogenic cells with non-muscle cells such as adipocytes, fibroblasts and vasculature are absent. The intimate cellular connection with ECM, which we now know is an important source of local growth factors and regulatory molecules, is lost in cell cultures. Contact with nerve cells, which play an important role in muscle growth, development and function, is also missing. Although cell cultures are a valuable tool to study growth factor effects on myogenesis, results must be interpreted with these limitations in mind.

Several types of muscle cell cultures are used to study myogenesis *in vitro*. Primary cultures of myogenic cells, derived from embryonic, fetal and postnatal muscle from a variety of species, have been used to study myogenesis. These cultures have a limited lifespan and, in general, cell isolates are prepared fresh for each experiment. While this may introduce individual animal variation into the experiment, many scientists believe that the cells used in primary cell cultures are more similar to those of the animal from which they are isolated. Myogenic cell lines are generally 'immortalized' by transformation to provide cells that grow continuously. Many cell lines are derived from cancerous cells that continuously replicate. Thus, cell lines often represent aberrant, continuously proliferating cell behaviour, respond differently to hormones and growth factors than non-transformed cells and express a different set of genes than non-transformed cells. Nevertheless, several myogenic cell lines have been used to study muscle development and these have provided insight into the regulatory mechanisms involved in myogenesis. These include the L6 myoblast cell line, derived from fetal rat thigh muscle, as well as clones from L6 cells, L6A1 and L6E9. The C2C12 clone of the C2 satellite cell line is derived from the adult mouse, as are the cell lines Sol8, from the soleus muscle, and the BC3H1 cell line.

Primary cell cultures and cell lines are used to study the processes of proliferation, differentiation and fusion of myogenic cells. Cell proliferation can be studied by the direct enumeration of cell numbers using a microscope or electronic counting, or by quantifying the incorporation of radioactive thymidine (either ^{14}C or ^{3}H) into DNA. Differentiation of myoblasts into myotubes (multinucleated myofibre precursors) can be measured microscopically, counting the number of multinucleated cells formed in response to a stimulus, or molecular markers of the differentiated state can be examined. The activity of the muscle-specific creatine kinase enzyme or the expression of the myosin mRNA or protein are often used as markers for muscle differentiation. New molecular biology methods are used to quantitate the changes in gene expression during differentiation of MRFs such as MyoD or myogenin.

Muscle Regulatory Factors (MRFs)

MRFs are transcription factors that induce commitment to the myogenic lineage and induce myofibre differentiation. Each MRF can induce the complete myogenic programme in non-skeletal muscle cell types, such as fibroblasts *in vitro*, resulting in the formation of skeletal muscle. The MRFs belong to the superfamily of over 400 bHLH transcription factors. In vertebrates, the MRF subfamily consists of four members: Myf5 (myogenic factor 5), MyoD (myogenic determination factor D), MRF4 and myogenin. When these transcription factors are activated, they form homodimers with themselves and heterodimers with other bHLH transcription factors called E proteins. After dimerization, the MRFs bind to nucleotide sequences in the promotor region of affected genes called Eboxes, with the sequence 5'-GAGCTG-3'. Binding of MyoD and Myf5 to E boxes induces local changes in the chromatin (chromatin remodelling) in the regulatory region of genes. This results in the activation of specific gene targets by MyoD and Myf5.

The MRFs are expressed sequentially during embryonic development. They appear first in the somites and later in myoblasts of the limb bud. The formation of somites during embryonic development occurs in an anterior to posterior fashion. Similarly, the development of the embryonic anterior (forelimb) limb buds occurs before the hind limbs. Accompanying these developmental events, MRF expression is first seen in the anterior somites and as development progresses, expression of MRFs is seen in the posterior somites. Likewise, the anterior limb buds express the MRFs before the posterior limb buds. The Myf5 gene is the first MRF to be expressed (Table 7.1). Myf5 occurs in the epaxial dermomyotome, where it is found first, at day 8 in the mouse embryo (21-day gestation). It is expressed throughout the entire myotome as development proceeds and is downregulated by day 10.5. Myogenic cells in the mouse limb bud express Myf5 between embryonic days 10 and 12.

Expression of MyoD begins at day 9.75 in the hypaxial portion of the somite and is seen throughout the somite by day 11 of development. Somitic expression of MyoD is maintained throughout the fetal life. Like Myf5, MyoD is expressed between days 10 and 12 in the limb bud. Myogenin expression in the somites begins at day 8.5 and continues throughout fetal

Table 7.1. MRF gene expression in mouse embryos.

MRF gene	Embryonic source	Embryonic day (21 days gestation)
Myf5	Somite	8–10.5
	Limb bud	10–12
Myogenin	Somite	8.5–21
	Limb bud	10.5–21
MRF4	Somite	9–11.5
	Myofibre	16–21
MyoD	Somite	9.75–21
	Limb bud	10–12

development. In the limb buds, myogenin expression begins at day 10.5. Myogenin gene expression ceases in the postnatal animal.

The gene expression of MRF4 occurs in a biphasic manner during two embryonic periods. It is first expressed from day 9 to day 11.5 in the somites, is downregulated, and then is re-expressed in differentiated muscle fibres beginning at day 16 and for the remainder of development. Expression of MRF4 persists in the postnatal animal, where it is the most abundant of the MRFs.

Effects of the MRFs on muscle development

The functions of the MRFs have been determined using knockout mice in which a specific MRF gene (or genes) is disrupted. The expression of MyoD and Myf5 provides an excellent example of biological redundancy during skeletal muscle differentiation. When the MyoD gene is deleted from embryos, the resulting animals are viable, able to reproduce and have no obvious skeletal muscle defects. Expression of myogenin and MRF4 is unaffected. Closer examination of the development of these MyoD-deficient mice showed that the migration of hypaxial myoblasts, but not epaxial myoblasts, was delayed by about 3.5 days. In addition, the expression of Myf5 mRNA is increased in the postnatal mouse in the absence of MyoD. These observations suggest that in the absence of MyoD, Myf5 expression fills a compensatory role that allows normal muscle development to proceed even in the absence of MyoD. On the other hand, when the Myf5 gene is deleted, the embryos are not viable, the distal portion of the ribs does not form and somite formation is delayed for 2 days. These events occur despite the observation that both MyoD are myogenin are expressed normally. No obvious skeletal muscle defects are observed in neonatal mice after the deletion of Myf5 gene and the expression of other MRFs is not altered. In contrast to the MyoD-deficient animals, in which hypaxial myoblast migration is delayed, the formation of epaxial musculature is delayed in Myf5 knockout mice. When both the Myf5 and MyoD genes are deleted, myoblasts and skeletal muscle are not formed. The neonatal mice are immobile and die immediately after birth.

Mice lacking the myogenin gene die soon after parturition. The animals have major skeletal muscle deficiencies throughout the body, reduced myofibre density and muscle mass, as well as spinal and rib deformities. The muscles primarily affected by the absence of myogenin are those of the hypaxial musculature, in which muscle fibres are scarce or absent. The numbers of myoblasts in myogenin knockout mice are equivalent to those in normal mice. Studies *in vivo* and *in vitro* demonstrate that myogenin expression is upregulated during myoblast differentiation and fusion. Together, these observations suggest that the primary effects of myogenin occur after myoblast formation and that myogenin is required for the terminal differentiation of myoblasts into myotubes and myofibres.

The effects of deletion of the MRF4 gene are complicated by its proximity to the Myf5 gene. These genes are contiguous in mice and deletion of the

MRF4 gene also affects the regulation of the Myf5 gene. This is because regulatory elements that affect the regulation of the Myf5 gene are scattered throughout the introns in the MRF4 and Myf5 gene complex. MRF4 knockouts die in the perinatal period with deficient epaxial myogenesis, intercostal muscles and rib anomalies. A defect in myotome formation is also seen between days 9 and 11, when MRF4 is first expressed during normal development. Expression of the other three MRFs is also reduced at day 10, but myogenesis is apparently normal by day 14. Postnatal expression of myogenin is increased in the MRF4 knockout mice, suggesting that myogenin may, in part, compensate for the absence of MRF4.

These elegant experiments demonstrate the importance of the MRFs in skeletal muscle development. MyoD and Myf5 play essential roles in the recruitment, migration and differentiation of the myogenic lineage. The lack of overt skeletal muscle defects in single gene knockouts indicates that the effects of MyoD and Myf5 are redundant and in the absence of one of these MRFs, the other one can compensate for its loss. In the absence of both factors, no myoblasts or skeletal muscle is formed. For these reasons, MyoD and Myf5 are considered to be the primary myogenic regulatory factors that are required for the determination of the myogenic lineage. Myogenin and MRF4 are secondary factors in the regulation of myogenesis, as their effects occur later in development. Myogenin acts in myoblasts to induce terminal differentiation while MRF4 affects mature myofibres in the embryo and postnatal animal. In addition, observations from the MyoD and Myf5 knockout mice suggest that MyoD and myogenin regulate epaxial muscle development and the combination of Myf5 and MRF4 regulates hypaxial muscle formation.

Although the primary actions of the MRFs are during the embryonic development of muscle, they may also have effects in the adult animal. In postnatal muscle, MRF4 is the most abundant of the MRFs, suggesting a possible role of MRF4 in the maintenance of the differentiated state of skeletal muscle. MyoD and myogenin expression in mature skeletal muscle occurs only at low levels. In adult rats, MyoD expression is restricted to fast glycolytic fibres while myogenin is found only in slow oxidative fibres. This suggests that MyoD and myogenin may have fibre-specific effects in adult animals.

Regulation of MRF expression

The expression of MRFs is regulated by several factors (Fig. 7.1). The earliest processes in the formation of specialized myogenic precursor cells in the somites and their subsequent migration are accompanied by the increased expression of a number of genes. The expression of MRFs in the somites is influenced by paracrine signals from adjacent tissues. For example, the embryonic notochord and the ventral neural tube secrete SHH, while morphogens from the wingless genes (wnts 1, 3 and 4) are secreted from the dorsal neural tube and ectoderm of the embryo. Along with SHH, wnt initiates dermomyotome formation and myogenic cell recruitment, by inducing

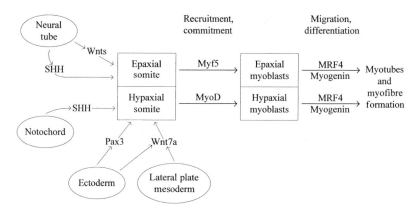

Fig. 7.1. Regulation of embryonic myogenesis by MRFs and morphogens.

MyoD and Myf5 and myogenin expression in the differentiating muscle cells. SHH induces the expression of Myf5 and MyoD in the dermomyotome and rapid differentiation and hypertrophy of skeletal muscle.

In the somites, the development of a muscle progenitor pool in the lateral dermomyotome is accompanied by the increased expression of the transcription factor Pax3 (Paired Box 3). Pax3 is first expressed at day 8.5 in the dermomyotome. The expression of Pax3 continues in the myoblasts migrating from the somite to the limb bud. Embryonic mice in which the Pax3 gene is deleted die before day 15 of development. In these animals, myogenic cells do not migrate from the somites to areas of muscle formation and there is an absence of muscles in the limbs, back and diaphragm. The expression of MyoD is under the dual control of Pax3 and Myf5. Although MyoD expression is not affected in the absence of Pax3, ablation of both Pax3 and Myf5 genes abolishes MyoD expression and skeletal muscle does not form.

Another transcription factor, Lbx1 (Ladybird homeobox 1), is involved in the delamination of lateral somite cells and is required for migration of somitic cells into the limb bud. Lbx1 is first expressed at day 8 in the dermomyotome and Lbx1 is found in migrating cells at day 10. Ablation of the Lbx1 gene leads to an absence or extreme reduction of limb muscles, as cells from the somite fail to migrate. In addition, HGF, and its tyrosine kinase receptor called c-Met, are involved in the migration of cells from the lateral somites to the limb buds. HGF is discussed in detail below.

Upon arrival in the limb bud, the myoblasts rapidly proliferate under the influence of FGF-2, -4 and -8, which are secreted by the ectoderm overlying the limb bud. Proliferation of the myoblasts increases cell numbers to provide additional sources of myoblasts while differentiation is delayed. The mesenchyme in the posterior margin of the limb bud, called the zone of polarizing activity, secretes the SHH, which is responsible for the anterior–posterior positioning of the limb and induction of myogenic factors that stimulate differentiation. Both FGF and SHH are required to coordinate limb formation and in the absence of either factor limb development ceases.

Growth Factors Affecting Muscle Growth

IGFs

The IGFs play a central role in the development, differentiation and mainte-nance of skeletal muscle (Fig. 7.2). The IGFs are produced by the liver as well as by cells of the skeletal muscle system, including myoblasts, satellite cells, myofibres and fibroblasts. Thus, these ubiquitous growth factors may act via endocrine, paracrine and autocrine pathways to affect skeletal muscle growth and metabolism. Current experimental data suggest that the effects of IGFs on muscle growth are primarily local autocrine and paracrine effects. With the exception of the C2C12 satellite cell line, there are few or no mus-cle GH receptors and, when studied *in vitro*, GH effects on muscle growth and differentiation cannot be demonstrated. This suggests that GH has no direct anabolic effects on myoblasts, satellite cells or myotubes and the observed effects of GH in the intact animal are probably due to locally pro-duced IGFs. In skeletal muscle, the IGFs increase glucose and amino acid uptake, decrease proteolysis and increase protein synthesis. In addition, they have effects on muscle precursor cells, increasing myoblast and satellite cell proliferation and differentiation. The IGFs are the only extracellular growth factors which are capable of inducing the terminal differentiation of myoblasts and satellite cells. The direct effects of IGFs on mature myofibres result in an induction of muscle hypertrophy of glycolytic, Type IIb fibres.

Most primary cell cultures and myogenic cell lines secrete and respond to IGFs, suggesting an autocrine mechanism of action. In addition, embry-onic and adult muscle cells express IGFs during development. In porcine embryos, the expression of muscle IGF-I and IGF-II genes increases during the latter phase of primary muscle fibre formation, from days 44 to 59 of ges-tation. During the time of secondary myofibre formation (day 75 and on) in pigs, expression of IGF-I is increased further while IGF-II expression steadily declines. These observations suggest that the IGFs play important regulatory roles in all phases of myogenesis *in vivo* and *in vitro*.

Administration of IGFs to experimental animals induces an increase in muscle mass while the removal of IGF reduces muscle mass. Knockout mice in which the IGF-I gene is deleted results in a phenotype similar to myo-genin knockout mice, with a generalized failure of skeletal muscle develop-ment. Similarly, Type I IGF receptor knockout mice are about half the size of wild-type mice and suffer from generalized muscle hypoplasia. Deletion of the Type II IGF receptor results in neonatal mice that are actually about 30% heavier than their normal littermates. These mice have elevated levels of IGF-II and die in the postnatal period. This suggests that the role of the Type II receptor is not to mediate the effects of IGF-II on muscle growth. Instead, this receptor is believed to act as a negative regulator of circulating IGF-II levels, internalizing IGF-II into cells and degrading it. This protects the ani-mal from excessively high levels of IGF-II.

Studies on myogenic cells *in vitro* show that the IGFs induce both prolif-eration and differentiation of myoblasts and satellite cells. Both IGF-I and

IGF-II are capable of myogenic regulation, but larger doses of IGF-II are required to induce the same effects as those seen with IGF-I. This supports the belief that the effects of IGF-II on muscle cells (as well as other cells) are mediated by the Type I IGF receptor or, possibly, the insulin receptor. As IGF-II has a lower affinity for these receptors than their primary ligands, higher concentrations of IGF-II are needed to induce muscle functions. Nevertheless, IGF-II may be more important than IGF-I for differentiation of skeletal muscle. IGF-II levels increase 20–30-fold during differentiation of myoblasts into myotubes, suggesting that autocrine effects of IGF-II are involved in skeletal muscle differentiation.

The effects of IGFs on myogenesis depend upon the stage of myoblast development. At early times of development, the IGFs stimulate proliferation. Sustained stimulation of cells by the IGFs leads to cellular differentiation, characterized by activation of myogenin, Myf5 and MyoD expression. In addition, the effects of IGFs on muscle cells are concentration-dependent. Low concentrations of IGF-I or IGF-II stimulate dose-dependent differentiation, while higher concentrations inhibit differentiation of myoblasts. These effects, seen in the artificial environment of cell culture *in vitro*, likely mimic physiological processes in the animal. Thus, a muscle cell is likely to be exposed to IGFs only during certain developmental stages that are regulated by specific, temporal IGF gene expression. Likewise, very high, localized concentrations of IGFs may be expected to be present in the ECM. Exposure of cells to these elevated levels as paracrine or autocrine signals is likely to induce different responses than seen with lower concentrations of IGFs.

Two different Type I IGF receptor-activated intracellular pathways mediate the effects of IGFs in myogenic cells. The effects of IGF-I on cell proliferation is believed to be mediated by the MAP kinase pathway while the PI-3 kinase pathway mediates the effects of IGF-I on muscle differentiation. Likewise, the IGFs have differential effects on the expression of the MRF genes during cell proliferation and differentiation. When cell proliferation is induced by the IGFs, MRF expression is inhibited and when myogenic differentiation is induced by the IGFs, MRF4 and myogenin gene expression are upregulated. When the myogenin gene mRNA is neutralized with antisense oligonucleotides, IGF-I treatment fails to induce differentiation. This indicates that myogenin expression is an obligatory event in the IGF-I induction of differentiation. When the Type I IGF receptor is deleted, myogenin and MyoD expression are delayed *in vivo* and *in vitro*, suggesting that activation of the IGF receptor is at least partially responsible for the induction of these genes. Thus, the IGFs play a central role in the induction of proliferation and differentiation of myogenic precursor cells, acting to induce or suppress MRF expression. These effects of IGFs result in an increase in myoblast and myofibre numbers.

In addition to the effects of IGFs on myogenic cell proliferation and differentiation, the IGFs play crucial roles in the induction and maintenance of mature skeletal muscle growth. Muscle hypertrophy is stimulated in transgenic mice in which the IGF-I gene is specifically expressed in skeletal muscle.

Transfection of myotubes with the IGF-I gene *in vitro* also induces cellular hypertrophy. In the intact animal, adult skeletal muscle growth is due to the addition of satellite cell nuclei to the amitotic myofibres. Several studies in multiple laboratories over the past 20 years have shown that the IGFs induce satellite cell proliferation, differentiation and fusion to form myotubes.

Effects of the IGFs on hypertrophy are accompanied by alterations in protein and carbohydrate metabolism. The IGFs stimulate amino acid uptake and protein synthesis while inhibiting protein degradation in a variety of myogenic cells *in vitro*, including myoblasts, satellite cells and myotubes. Treatment of mice with IGF-I also stimulates protein synthesis and inhibits protein degradation in skeletal muscle. The metabolic energy that is used for muscle hypertrophy, protein synthesis and contraction is derived from the oxidation of glucose. One of the early bioassays for IGFs involved the IGF-stimulated oxidation of glucose by isolated adipose tissue. In muscle cells, IGFs also stimulate glucose uptake and oxidation.

Myostatin

Myostatin, also known as GDF-8, is a secreted growth factor that is a member of the TGF-β superfamily. Myostatin is a 15 kDa peptide with autocrine and paracrine actions in skeletal muscle. The myostatin molecule is highly conserved between a wide range of species, and is identical in mice, rats, humans, pigs and birds. This molecular conservation suggests that myostatin is an evolutionarily conserved essential factor that plays a central role in physiological processes that are common to a wide spectrum of animals. Myostatin is expressed in cells very early in embryonic development and is present in chick blastoderm, the avian equivalent of the mammalian blastocyst. It is also expressed later in embryogenesis, when it appears in the dermomyotome of the somites. In addition, myostatin is expressed in the adult, and is found in satellite cells and mature myofibres. Myostatin is not restricted to skeletal muscle, and is also present in adipose tissue and the mammary gland.

In contrast to many of the growth and transcription factors that regulate myogenesis, myostatin is a negative regulator of muscle growth. Although many growth factors delay differentiation by increasing proliferation, the TGF-β superfamily of peptides, including BMP, TGF-β and myostatin, reduce cell proliferation rates and, thus, delay differentiation. Myostatin inhibits myogenic differentiation by inhibiting the expression of the myogenic transcription factors MyoD and myogenin. When myoblasts are treated with myostatin, cell proliferation, DNA and protein synthesis are reduced. In contrast, when muscle atrophy is induced by denervation, the synthesis of myostatin protein and mRNA is upregulated in the muscle fibres. This indicates that myogenin plays a significant role in the activation and recruitment of satellite cells that are responsible for the regeneration of the atrophied muscle. The myostatin gene is expressed in proliferating satellite cells *in vitro*, and its expression increases prior to myotube formation. Thus, myostatin may be a major factor that activates satellite cells during muscle hypertrophy and regeneration. This is further supported by studies in knockout mice, in which deletion of the myostatin gene stimulates satellite cell division, skeletal muscle hypertrophy and a two- to threefold increase in muscle mass.

A naturally occurring mutation of the bovine myostatin gene has been identified that results in an inactive myostatin molecule. This has been shown to be the cause of the muscle hypertrophy that results in the so-called double-muscled phenotype in cattle breeds. Although these animals do not have twice the number of muscles as other breeds, they are characterized by excessive musculature due to hypertrophy. Cattle breeds such as the Belgian Blue, Piedmontese and Asturiana de la Valle result from mutational inactivation of the myostatin molecule. Interestingly, a human infant has recently been identified with a myostatin mutation. This child displays the excessive musculature and muscular hypertrophy characteristic of myostatin deficiency.

FGF

FGF is a potent inhibitor of muscle differentiation but plays a key role in early myoblast development. FGF has both autocrine and paracrine effects on developing muscle cells. The FGF gene is expressed in the early embryonic somite and later in development in the overlying ectoderm of the limb bud. After synthesis and secretion, FGF is stored in the ECM, where it is bound to heparin sulphate and Syndecan3. FGF mRNA and protein are found in proliferating satellite cells, myoblasts and macrophages. FGF receptors are present in myoblasts and satellite cells, but are absent in myotubes. FGF inhibits differentiation by stimulating mitosis of myoblasts and satellite cells, thereby delaying differentiation. In proliferating myogenic cells, FGF suppresses the expression of the MRFs, MyoD and myogenin. This inhibits MRF induction of the specific myogenic genes needed for muscle differentiation. FGF increases chemotaxis of stem cells and stimulates angiogenesis, the formation of new blood vessels for tissue growth. FGF inhibits the expression of IGF-II and may block some of the effects of IGF-II on myogenic differentiation. If the effects of FGF are blocked in myoblasts by receptor mutations, myoblasts differentiate prematurely into myofibres. As a result, there is a 30% reduction in limb muscle weight and a 50% reduction in muscle fibre numbers in these animals. This demonstrates the importance of FGF in myogenesis, a factor that has an inhibitory effect on muscle differentiation, but one that is essential to provide adequate numbers of myoblasts to form normal musculature.

TGF-β

Like FGF, TGF-β is a potent inhibitor of muscle differentiation. Many cells produce TGF-β, including myoblasts and regenerating muscle tissue. After secretion, TGF-β is stored in the ECM bound to the protein decorin. The main iso-form of TGF-β found in skeletal muscle is TGF-β3. It has been shown that TGF-β inhibits the differentiation of myogenic cells. It does this by slowing the proliferation of myoblasts and satellite cells. As was the case with FGF, TGF-β treatment inhibits the expression of MyoD and myogenin in myogenic cells. In addition TGF-β3 has distinct effects on the ECM, inducing the synthesis of collagen and fibronectin. Overall, TGF-β is an important inhibitor of the terminal differentiation of skeletal muscle, while ensuring that there is an adequate precursor pool of undifferentiated, quiescent myogenic cells. Coincidentally, TGF-β induces angiogenesis of developing tissues, providing the vascular supply needed for muscle growth and development.

BMPs

The BMPs, members of the TGF-β family, have distinct effects during skeletal muscle differentiation. In the embryo, cells of the ectoderm, mesoderm and the neural tube produce the BMPs that act on adjacent myogenic cells in the somites and the limb bud. BMP4 functions in mesodermal cell determination into the myogenic line and formation of myoblasts. Like other members of the TGF-β family, BMP4 slows myoblast proliferation and prevents premature myoblast differentiation in the somites.

Hepatocyte growth factor

HGF was initially characterized as a potent mitogen for hepatocytes. It is identical to 'scatter factor', named because of its stimulatory effects on epithelial cell motility. It has since been shown to be mitogenic for many endothelial and epithelial cells. HGF is an autocrine and paracrine mediator of morphogenesis in the myogenic cell lineage and is also important in the development of the liver and placenta. The HGF molecule consists of a disulphide-linked heterodimer with a molecular weight of 70 to 80 kDa. HGF is secreted as a large monomer that is activated by proteolytic removal of a portion of the precursor molecule. Secreted HGF is stored in the ECM of skeletal muscle. Heparin sulphate of the ECM is required for the HGF activation of the HGF receptor. The effects of HGF are mediated by the cell surface tyrosine kinase receptor, c-Met.

HGF plays a central role in the initial events that trigger the myogenic cascade. HGF induces the initial conversion of epithelial cells in the somite into mesenchymal cells, establishing the somitic pool of myogenic precursor cells. This epithiomesenchymal conversion is accompanied by the assumption of mesenchymal cell motility and migration of myoblasts from the somite to areas of hypaxial muscle formation. Along with the transcription factors Lbx1 and Pax3, HGF mediates myoblast delamination from the dermomyotome and myoblast migration to sites of muscle formation. The delamination and migration of myoblasts from the somite to the developing limb bud is stimulated by paracrine HGF, which is secreted by mesenchymal cells along the routes of myoblast migration and by limb bud mesenchyme. When HGF or the HGF receptor (c-Met) gene is inactivated, hypaxial myoblast migration fails, and skeletal muscles in the limb and diaphragm do not form, although epaxial skeletal muscle is not affected. As this migratory failure occurs despite continued Lbx1 expression, HGF and its receptor are believed to be the primary inducers of myoblast delamination, migration and colonization of sites of muscle formation.

HGF has also been shown to be involved in adult muscle hypertrophy and regeneration. Muscle regeneration in response to physical trauma or exercise essentially recapitulates the embryonic myogenic pathway. Quiescent satellite cells are activated, proliferate, differentiate and fuse into contractile myotubes *in vitro*. In animals, satellite cells fuse with myofibres and provide new nuclei at local sites for muscle repair and hypertrophy. HGF is the first growth factor to activate satellite cell proliferation, ending the dormant state and inducing satellite cell entry into the cell cycle and mitosis. HGF is synthesized and secreted by primary cultures of chicken and turkey satellite cells and the C2 satellite cell line, and HGF is restricted to satellite cells and the surrounding ECM. HGF is not detected in muscle-derived fibroblasts or myofibres. As satellite cells express the c-Met HGF receptor, HGF is believed to act via an autocrine pathway to activate quiescent satellite cells. Expression of the c-Met receptor in satellite cells declines during differentiation. HGF effects on satellite cells are mediated by an inhibition of expression of the bHLH transcription factors, MyoD and myogenin. The regulation of myogenesis by growth factors is shown in Fig. 7.2.

Hormones regulating muscle growth

The role of hormones that directly regulate the growth and development of skeletal muscle is relatively limited. As discussed in detail in the current and preceding chapters, GH plays an important, albeit indirect, role in the development of skeletal muscle, with its actions mediated by the IGFs. As discussed in previous chapters, the steroids and the catecholamine-derived β-agonists provide important tools in the regulation of farm animal muscle growth. Other hormones, such as insulin, thyroid hormones and glucocorticoids, play a primarily permissive role in the growth, differentiation and maintenance of muscle.

Insulin is required to maintain adequate cellular energy supply, by maintaining a constant concentration of serum glucose and by regulating cellular glucose uptake, an essential component of normal cell growth and metabolism. In the animal, insulin stimulates the deposition of glycogen, protein and triglycerol, acting in concert with other anabolic and catabolic hormones. Insulin has no effects on brain glucose uptake and the gut and skin are largely insensitive to insulin. Insulin also stimulates amino acid transport, protein synthesis and inhibits protein degradation during tissue growth. Although insulin is essential for protein accretion, insulin treatment

Stem cells – pluripotent mesoderm

↓   *Determination*: HGF, IGF, SHH

Myoblasts and satellite cells (SCs activated by HGF/c-Met)

↓   *Determination*: HGF

↓   *Proliferation*: FGF, PDGF, TGF-β (–), IGF

↓   *Differentiation*: IGFs, myogenin/MRF4

↓   *Fusion*: IGF, HGF

Myotubes

↓   *Fusion, hypertrophy*: IGF, FGF, HGF

Myofibres

Fig. 7.2. The role of growth factors in the regulation of myogenesis.

of animals does not produce positive results, due to insulin induction of hypoglycaemia. In postnatal skeletal muscle, insulin has anabolic effects. Individuals with diabetes mellitus suffer from muscle wasting, a condition that is reversed by insulin treatment. The effects of insulin on growth and differentiation of myogenic cells requires very high, pharmacological doses of insulin. For example, insulin induces growth and differentiation of satellite cells, myoblasts and fibroblasts when 1 µM insulin is present. This is an extremely high dose of insulin, equivalent to ~5 mg/ml, a concentration never achieved in the animal. The effects of insulin on myogenic growth and differentiation are probably due to cross-reaction with the Type I IGF receptor at high concentrations of insulin.

Adrenal glucocorticoids are generally considered to inhibit growth. Glucocorticoids are considered as glucose-sparing hormones that reduce glucose use by tissues, increase gluconeogenesis and induce hyperglycaemia. These effects are in opposition to those seen with insulin, and glucocorticoids provide a balance to the effects of insulin on glucose metabolism. Physiological doses of glucocorticoids inhibit cell replication and protein synthesis in a variety of cell types *in vitro*. *In vivo*, glucocorticoid treatment of animals slows growth and inhibits the secretion of GH and the IGFs. Protein catabolism by muscle is increased by glucocorticoids, *in vivo* and *in vitro*. This results in a reduced incorporation of amino acids into muscle protein and an increased release of amino acids by muscle. Long-term or high-dose treatment of animals induces muscle atrophy. Nevertheless, glucocorticoids, in the form of synthetic dexamethasone, are often added to myogenic cell culture medium. In the artificial environment in which cells are grown *in vitro*, the presence of glucocorticoids provides a counter-regulatory effect for the anabolic actions of other factors (e.g. insulin) to ensure adequate balance between intracellular and extracellular glucose homeostasis.

It has long been known that a deficiency of thyroid hormones, either from a dysfunctional thyroid or an absence of dietary iodine, leads to growth retardation. Thyroid hormones play important roles in the development of the CNS and neonatal and pre-pubertal deficiencies in thyroid hormones result in reduced CNS myelination, mental retardation and the syndrome known as cretinism in humans. Thyroid hormones are largely permissive agents for muscle growth and differentiation. Along with GH and growth factors, thyroid hormones are required for normal muscle development. Thyroid hormones stimulate the synthesis of protein and RNA in skeletal muscle and are important in maturation of skeletal muscle. As neonatal rat muscle matures, myosin shifts from a slow, embryonic isoform to a fast twitch, adult isoform. This transition is accelerated by thyroid hormones and is retarded in hypothyroid animals. The primary metabolic effect of thyroid hormones is to stimulate energy use, oxidative metabolism and metabolic rate. Exposure of animals to high doses of thyroid hormones induces protein degradation and muscle atrophy. The effects of thyroid hormones on energy metabolism and muscle atrophy, which predominate in long-term or high-dose treatments, preclude the use of thyroid hormones as growth promotants.

Further Reading

Allen, R.E. and Boxhorn, L.K. (1989) Regulation of skeletal muscle satellite cell proliferation and differentiation by transforming growth factor-beta, insulin-like growth factor I, and fibroblast growth factor. *Journal of Cellular Physiology* 138, 311–315.

Allen, R.E., Sheehan, S.M., Taylor, R.G., Kendall, T.L. and Rice, G.M. (1995) Hepatocyte growth factor activates quiescent skeletal muscle satellite cells *in vitro*. *Journal of Cellular Physiology* 165, 307–312.

Atchley, W.R. and Fitch, W.M. (1997) A natural classification of the basic helix–loop–helix class of transcription factors. *Proceedings of the National Academy of the Sciences USA* 94, 5172–5176.

Borycki, A.G. and Emerson, C.P. Jr. (2000) Multiple tissue interactions and signal transduction pathways control somite myogenesis. *Current Topics in Developmental Biology* 48, 165–224.

Borycki, A.G., Brunk, B., Tajbakhsh, S., Buckingham, M., Chiang, C. and Emerson, C.P. Jr. (1999) Sonic hedgehog controls epaxial muscle determination through Myf5 activation. *Development* 126, 4053–4063.

Brand-Saberi, B. (ed.) (2002) Vertebrate myogenesis. In: *Results and Problems in Cell Differentiation*, Vol. 38. Springer-Verlag, New York, 242 pp.

Brohmann, H., Jagla, K. and Birchmeier, C. (2000) The role of Lbx1 in migration of muscle precursor cells. *Development* 127, 437–445.

Florini, J.R. and Ewton, D.Z. (1988) Actions of transforming growth factor-beta on muscle cells. *Journal of Cellular Physiology* 135, 301–308.

Florini, J.R., Ewton, D.Z., Falen, S.L. and Van Wyk, J.J. (1986) Biphasic concentration dependence of stimulation of myoblast differentiation by somatomedins. *American Journal of Physiology* 250, C771–C778.

Florini, J.R., Ewton, D.Z., Magri, K.A. and Mangiacapra, F.J. (1994) IGFs and muscle differentiation. In: LeRoith, D. and Raizada, M.K. (eds) *Current Directions in Insulin-like Growth Factor Research*. Plenum Press, New York, pp. 319–326.

Hasty, P., Bradley, A., Morris, J.H., Edmondson, D.G., Venuti, J.M., Olson, E.N. and Klein, W.H. (1993) Muscle deficiency and neonatal death in mice with a targeted mutation in the myogenin gene. *Nature* 364, 501–506.

Kablar, B., Krastel, K., Ying, C., Tapscott, S.J., Goldhamer, D.J. and Rudnicki, M.A. (1999) Myogenic determination occurs independently in somites and limb buds. *Developmental Biology* 206, 219–231.

Kaul, A., Koster, M., Neuhaus, H. and Braun, T. (2000) Myf-5 revisited: loss of early myotome formation does not lead to a rib phenotype in homozygous Myf-5 mutant mice. *Cell* 102, 17–19.

Kocamis, H. and Killefer, J. (2002) Myostatin expression and possible functions in animal muscle growth. *Domestic Animal Endocrinology* 23, 447–454.

Milasincic, D.J., Calera, M.R., Farmer, S.R. and Pilch, P.F. (1996) Stimulation of C2C12 myoblast growth by basic fibroblast growth factor and insulin-like growth factor 1 can occur via mitogen-activated protein kinase-dependent and -independent pathways. *Molecular and Cellular Biology* 16, 5964–5973.

Molkentin, J.D. and Olson, E.N. (1996) Defining the regulatory networks for muscle development. *Current Opinion in Genetics and Development* 6, 445–453.

Oksbjerg, N., Gondret, F. and Vestergaard, M. (2004) Basic principles of muscle development and growth in meat-producing mammals as affected by the insulin-like growth factor (IGF) system. *Domestic Animal Endocrinology* 27, 219–240.

Olson, E.N., Arnold, H.H., Rigby, P.W. and Wold, B.J. (1996) Know your neighbors: three phenotypes in null mutants of the myogenin bHLH gene MRF4. *Cell* 85, 1–4.

Olwin, B.B., Bren-Mattison, Y., Cornelison, D.D.W., Federov, Y.V., Flanagan-Steet, H. and Jones, N.C. (2002) Role of cytokines in skeletal muscle growth and differentiation. In: Sassoon, D.A. (ed.) *Advances in Developmental Biology and Biochemistry*. Vol. 11. *Stem Cells and Cell Signalling in Skeletal Myogenesis*. Elsevier, Amsterdam, pp. 97–126.

Palmer, C.M. and Rudnicki, M.A. (2002) The myogenic regulatory factors. In: Sassoon, D.A. (ed.) *Advances in Developmental Biology and Biochemistry*, Vol. 11. *Stem Cells and Cell Signalling in Skeletal Myogenesis*. Elsevier, Amsterdam, pp. 1–32.

Rawls, A. and Olson, E.N. (1997) MyoD meets its maker. *Cell* 89, 5–8.

Rios, R., Carneiro, I., Arce, V.M. and Devesa, J. (2002) Myostatin is an inhibitor of myogenic differentiation. *American Journal of Physiology. Cell Physiology* 282, C993–C999.

Rudnicki, M.A., Schnegelsberg, P.N., Stead, R.H., Braun, T., Arnold, H.H. and Jaenisch, R. (1993) MyoD or Myf-5 is required for the formation of skeletal muscle. *Cell* 75, 1351–1359.

Tajbakhsh, T. and Buckingham, M. (2000) The birth of muscle progenitor cells in the mouse: spatiotemporal considerations. *Current Topics in Developmental Biology* 48, 225–268.

Valdez, M.R., Richardson, J.A., Klein, W.H. and Olson, E.N. (2000) Failure of Myf5 to support myogenic differentiation without myogenin, MyoD and MRF4. *Developmental Biology* 219, 287–298.

Webb, S.E. and Lee, K.K. (1997) Effect of platelet-derived growth factor iso-forms on the migration of mouse embryo limb myogenic cells. *The International Journal of Developmental Biology* 41, 597–605.

Zhu, X., Hadhazy, M., Wehling, M., Tidball, J.G. and McNally, E.M. (2000) Dominant negative myostatin produces hypertrophy without hyperplasia in muscle. *FEBS Letters* 474, 71–75.

8 Hormones, Growth Factors and Adipose Tissue

This chapter is devoted to the control of growth and differentiation of adipose tissue by hormones and growth factors. Like bone, adipose tissue is classified histologically as a connective tissue. In contrast with most organs, adipose tissue is present not in a single location, but is spread throughout the body in many sites. White adipose tissue is an energy-dense tissue that serves as a nutrient depot for the body, a tissue that stores energy in the form of triacylglycerols in times of excess caloric intake. In times of nutrient deficiency lipid reserves stored in white adipose tissue are mobilized to provide metabolic energy to the animal. In contrast, brown adipose tissue is a specialized type of fat involved with cold adaptation and the generation of heat to maintain body temperature. This chapter deals primarily with white adipose tissue. Recently, adipose tissue has been shown to be a dynamic tissue that secretes a variety of factors that are actively involved in the regulation of such diverse processes as appetite, metabolism, the immune response, reproduction and haematopoiesis. These newly discovered functions expand the role of adipose tissue to that of an endocrine organ that secretes a variety of hormones and growth factors. The fundamental differentiation and development of adipose have been examined in Chapter 4. The primary goal of this chapter is to examine the hormones, growth factors and transcription factors that control adipose tissue development and maintain adipose tissue function. In addition, the role of adipose tissue as an endocrine organ will be discussed.

Cell Systems Used to Study Adipogenesis

Because of the diffuse nature of adipose tissue depots and the difficulties with examining a small population of undifferentiated preadipocytes in the whole animal, most studies examining the differentiation of adipocytes are performed using enriched preadipocyte cell preparations *in vitro*. Preadipocytes are present in the stromovascular cell fraction of adipose tissue and primary cell cultures derived from the stromovascular cell fraction can be used to study differentiation into adipocytes. The stromovascular fraction of adipose tissue contains fibroblasts, endothelial cells and stromal cells. These cells cannot be distinguished morphologically or biochemically from the presumptive preadipocytes in the stromovascular fraction, but may provide paracrine agents and a cellular environment more akin to the situation *in vivo*. The presence of preadipocytes in primary cultures can be distinguished from other cell types only by *post hoc* analysis. That is, only after differentiation and the expression of differentiation-specific molecular markers or formation of the lipid-containing adipocyte phenotype can the presence of the precursor preadipocyte cell be deduced.

The use of primary cell cultures of adipocytes, like those of any tissue, has the advantage that the cells are isolated from 'normal' animals using the species of choice. This is very important when studies about adipocyte metabolism from farm animals are undertaken, as these cells are available only from isolated primary cell cultures. Primary tissue culture cells are not transformed into immortalized cells capable of continuous replication *in vitro* and they are thus believed to be more similar to the cells seen in the intact animal than those of cell lines. A disadvantage of using primary cells is that the cells do not survive over a long period of time *in vitro*, and must be isolated anew for each experiment. This involves a great deal of labour and expense and introduces individual animal variation into the analysis.

An alternative to using primary cell cultures is the use of established preadipocyte cell lines. Pluripotent mouse fibroblast cell lines, such as the C3H10T1/2 and the NIH 3T3 cell lines, are capable of differentiation into preadipocytes and adipocytes. Clones of the mouse embryonic NIH 3T3 fibroblasts, denoted 3T3-L1 and 3T3-F442A, are preadipocyte cell lines that are committed to the adipogenic lineage and undergo differentiation into adipocytes under appropriate hormonal treatment. These cell lines have provided invaluable tools to study adipose cell differentiation and provided much of our current knowledge about the cellular and molecular regulation of adipogenesis. The advantages of using cell lines are that they can be cultured easily and grown continuously *in vitro*. On the other hand, as these cells are usually derived from embryonic or tumourigenic sources, they may not display the physiological characteristics or responses to stimuli that affect primary cell cultures isolated from normal animals. The 3T3 cell lines also suffer from aneuploidy, a state in which chromosome numbers are not an exact multiple of the original chromosome number of the animal from which they are derived. This may alter their physiological characteristics and responses to external stimuli. Cells grown in monolayers *in vitro* also suffer from a lack of three-dimensional organization seen in the animal and lack their normal extracellular support and interactions with surrounding lipogenic and non-lipogenic cells. The available cell lines differentiate into white adipose tissue. Cell lines for the study of brown adipose tissue are not available. In addition, available cell lines are usually derived from human or rodent sources and may have no relevance to domestic animal physiology. Preadipocyte cell lines for specific species, such as ruminants, do not exist.

The process of 3T3-L1 preadipocyte differentiation follows an ordered, repeatable sequence of events that can be reliably studied *in vitro* (Fig. 8.1).

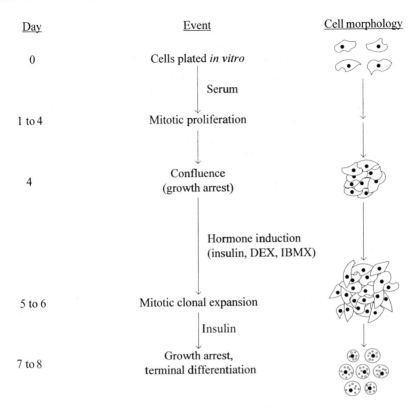

Day	Event	Cell morphology
0	Cells plated *in vitro*	
	Serum	
1 to 4	Mitotic proliferation	
4	Confluence (growth arrest)	
	Hormone induction (insulin, DEX, IBMX)	
5 to 6	Mitotic clonal expansion	
	Insulin	
7 to 8	Growth arrest, terminal differentiation	

Fig. 8.1. The differentiation of 3T3-L1 cells.

Most of our knowledge of the processes involved with adipocyte differentiation, gene expression and hormonal regulation of these processes has been gained from this system. Similar processes occur when preadipocytes isolated from stromovascular cells are studied *in vitro*. After cells are put into culture, they are maintained in a growth medium supplemented with mammalian serum. This provides the cells with nutrients and growth factors needed to induce a mitotic state and cells undergo proliferation. After the cells have replicated to the point of confluence, that is, when they cover the entire culture plate, they exit the cell cycle and become quiescent. They are then transferred to a culture medium supplemented with a hormone cocktail that induces differentiation into adipocytes during a 4-day period. Preadipocyte differentiation is stimulated by a medium containing a hormonal mixture of insulin or IGF-I, a glucocorticoid such as dexamethasone and isobutylmethylxanthine (IBMX). IBMX is a chemical that inhibits phosphodiesterase, the enzyme responsible for cAMP breakdown. Thus, the addition of IBMX increases cellular cAMP concentrations, and in the presence of dexamethasone and insulin, induces differentiation into lipid-filled adipocytes. The addition of this hormone cocktail induces the cells to re-enter the cell cycle and undergo one or two rounds of mitosis. This renewed mitotic behaviour is called clonal expansion. After exposure to this hormonal cocktail for 2 days, it is replaced by a medium containing only insulin. This induces the cells to withdraw from the cell cycle and begin the final process of terminal differentiation into adipocytes. After the 4-day hormonal induction period, more than 90% of the cells have assumed the adipocyte phenotype.

As with any cell studied *in vitro*, preadipocyte cell replication can be studied by measuring the incorporation of radioactive thymidine into nuclear DNA or by counting the number of cells that result from an experimental treatment. More sophisticated analyses monitor the expression of cell cycle-specific transcription factors to reflect the induction of mitosis. Differentiation of preadipocytes into mature adipocytes involves changes in the expression of over 2000 genes. The expression of some of these genes, either as protein or mRNA, can be quantitated and used as markers for assumption of the differentiated state. A few prominent molecular markers that are used to assess the differentiated state in adipocytes include genes expressed early in differentiation such as LPL, α-collagen VI and fatty acid transporter. Later markers of adipocyte differentiation include leptin, glycerol-3-phosphate dehydrogenase (GPDH), FAS, lipid-binding protein (ap2) and adipsin.

Transcription Factors and Adipogenesis

Cell differentiation is regulated by differential gene transcription. The differentiation of cells involves the shift of the gene expression pattern of cells from those genes associated with the pluripotent state of the primitive progenitor cells to an expression pattern seen in the differentiated cells. This is accompanied by morphological changes in the cell that arise as a consequence of altered gene expression. For example, during the differentiation of adipocytes, cell morphology changes from an irregular fibroblast-like shape to a cell that is rounded and begins to accumulate lipid. Changes in the hormonal and growth factor environment induce the expression of transcription factor genes that induce changes in adipocyte-specific gene expression and, subsequently, morphological and functional transformations.

Several transcription factors modulate adipose cell growth and differentiation. They are expressed sequentially in a time-specific, but overlapping manner by differentiating preadipocytes and terminally differentiated adipocytes. Many of them act in synergy with each other, enhancing one another's effects and inducing each other's expression. The cell system used most frequently to study these changes is the 3T3-L1 preadipocyte cell line, described earlier. With few exceptions, this model system is the basis for the following discussion of adipogenesis, as studied *in vitro*. The transcription factors that drive adipocyte differentiation are not expressed during the initial cell proliferation and confluence induced by serum. The transcription factors appear only after the addition of the hormone cocktail that reactivates the confluent cell cultures and initiates the differentiation programme of these cells. The transcription factors act at the level of the gene to induce or repress the expression of specific genes that regulate adipocyte differentiation and maintain the differentiated state. There are three major families of transcription factors that regulate adipocyte differentiation. These are peroxisome proliferator-activated receptor (PPAR), the C/EBP and the adipocyte determination and differentiation factor 1/sterol regulatory element-binding protein 1 (ADD1/SREBP1).

PPARs

As their name implies, the PPARs were first discovered as gene products that were induced by agents that stimulate peroxisome proliferation. Peroxisomes are intracellular, membrane-bound organelles, similar to lysosomes, that are present in all plant and animal cells. They are abundant in liver cells, where they occupy about 1% of the cell volume. Enzymes within the peroxisomes use oxygen as an oxidizing source and produce hydrogen peroxide (H_2O_2) as a by-product. In the liver, they play important roles in amino acid, uric acid and ethanol oxidation. Peroxisomes are also very important in the degradation of long-chain fatty acids via the β-oxidation pathway. This results in the formation of acetyl-CoA and H_2O_2.

The PPAR family of transcription factors plays a central role in the induction of the adipocyte differentiation programme. The potency of the PPARs in induction of adipogenesis is illustrated by the observation that PPARs can stimulate the differentiation of myoblasts into adipocytes and can induce the commitment of pluripotent fibroblasts, such as the C3H10T1/2 cell line, into the adipogenic cell lineage. The PPARs belong to the nuclear hormone receptor family. These receptors are activated by ligand binding to form heterodimers with other nuclear hormone receptors, the retinol X receptors (RXR). Formation of PPAR/RXR dimers induces binding of the complex to specific DNA sequences in the PPAR response elements. The specific sequences are called the DR-1 site and these are present in the promoter region of specific genes. Binding of the PPARs to the DR-1 sequences activates the transcription of genes that induce adipose differentiation and lipid synthesis.

The PPARs exist as three isoforms, PPARα, PPARδ (also called PPARβ) and PPARγ that share a high degree of amino acid homology in the two molecular domains that bind DNA and ligands. Despite these close homologies, the PPARs display distinct ligand specificity and DNA-binding sites. Ligands for the PPARs include long-chain fatty acids, fatty acid metabolites and drugs like the thiazolidinediones (TZDs) that reduce circulating lipid concentrations. The TZDs are some of the most important and widely studied of the PPARγ ligands. They are synthetic drugs that were developed for treatment of Type II (insulin-resistant) diabetes, as they reduce hyperlipidaemia and increase insulin sensitivity. It was only later that these drugs were found to be high affinity ligands for PPARγ and potent inducers of adipocyte differentiation. Most naturally occurring ligands for PPARγ are arachidonic acid derivatives such as prostaglandin D2 and the prostaglandin J2 metabolite, 15-deoxy-$\Delta^{12,14}$-prostaglandin J2.

The members of the PPAR family have different adipogenic activity, based on their potencies to induce 3T3-L1 cell differentiation into adipocytes. PPARα has only low adipogenic activity, PPARδ has no adipogenic activity while PPARγ is the most potent member of this family in the induction of the adipogenic lineage. PPARα occurs only at low levels in white adipose tissue but is present in high concentrations in brown adipose tissue. The adipogenic role of PPARα in white adipose tissue is believed to be minor and PPARα may be more important in the regulation of lipid metabolism. Mice in which the PPARα gene is disrupted have normal adipose tissue development, but display reduced β-oxidation of lipids in peroxisomes. The second member of the PPAR family, PPARδ, is found in many tissues in addition to adipocytes and its role, if any, in adipose cell differentiation is controversial and unclear.

PPARγ is the most potent of the PPAR family in the induction of adipocyte differentiation. It is the master regulator of adipocyte differentiation and adipocyte metabolism. It is the most abundant of the PPARs, occurring in adipose at levels that are 30-fold higher than in other tissues. PPARγ is the most fat-specific of the PPAR family. It is found in adipose tissue and adipocyte cell lines, but absent or present only in low levels in other tissues. Two forms of PPARγ, PPARγ1 and PPARγ2, result from alternate splicing of mRNA and alternate promoter sites of the PPARγ gene. PPARγ1 expression is widespread and is found in many different tissues, while PPARγ2 is found mainly in adipocytes. This suggests that PPARγ2 may have a more important role in adipocytes than PPARγ1, but this suggestion has not been adequately explored.

Expression of the PPARγ gene occurs early in adipogenesis, beginning about 1.5 days after hormone treatment of 3T3-L1 cells and persisting throughout terminal differentiation (Fig. 8.2). Overexpression of the PPARγ gene in preadipocytes induces the entire differentiated adipocyte phenotype, including the typical rounded adipocyte cell shape, lipid accumulation and the development of insulin sensitivity. PPARγ-induced differentiation of these cells is accompanied by the expression of adipocyte-specific genes such as fatty acid-binding protein (ap2), LPL, acetyl-coenzyme A carboxylase, leptin, FAS and SCD-1. In addition to its role in adipogenesis, PPARγ is also thought to be responsible for maintenance of the differentiated state of adipocytes. PPARγ is expressed in mature adipocytes and the PPAR response element is present in the genes for several lipogenic enzymes, including LPL, PEPCK and SCD.

Ligands which bind to and activate PPARγ include arachidonic acid metabolites, some polyunsaturated fatty acids (linoleic acid), the TZD drugs and non-steroidal anti-inflammatory drugs (NSAIDs). The binding affinity of the naturally occurring ligands for PPARγ is quite low, in the micromolar range. This contrasts with the high affinity (nanomolar) of the TZDs for PPARγ. The low affinity of currently identified PPARγ ligands casts doubt on their role in the physiological activation of PPARγ and the identity of

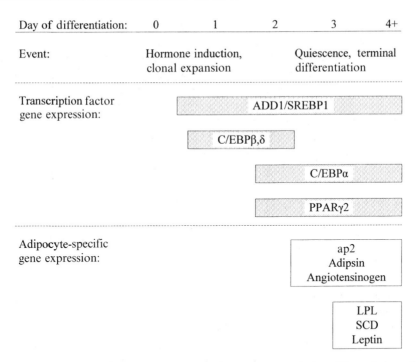

Fig. 8.2. Expression of transcription factors and adipocyte genes during differentiation of 3T3-L1 cells.

endogenous ligands for PPARγ is still uncertain. PPARγ is inactivated by phosphorylation of specific amino acid residues in the PPARγ molecule. Activation of the intracellular MAP kinase pathway inhibits adipogenesis. This has been shown to be due to the phosphorylation of PPARγ and RXR, which inhibits their activity.

C/EBPs

The C/EBP transcription factors are members of the basic leucine zipper family of transcription factors. The C/EBPs form homo- or heterodimer complexes with other molecules and bind to the CCAAT enhancer elements of gene regulatory sequences. The C/EBP are not limited to fat cells. They also play a role in the differentiation of hepatocytes and granulocyte cells of blood. There are six isoforms of the C/EBP molecules, which are formed by the use of differential transcription start sites on the C/EBP genes.

The primary C/EBP isoforms are C/EBPα, C/EBPβ and C/EBPδ. C/EBPβ and C/EBPδ mRNA and protein appear in 3T3-L1 cells about 12 h after hormone treatment and the expression of these genes subsides after 2 days (Fig. 8.2). The expression of C/EBPα begins after about 1.5 days of hormone treatment, just before terminal differentiation and the initiation of adipocyte-specific gene expression. C/EBPα expression persists in the differentiated adipocytes throughout the culture period.

The functional roles of the C/EBPs have been studied using transgenic mice and cell lines and in mice in which the C/EBP gene has been disrupted. Ectopic expression of the gene for C/EBPα or C/EBPβ in 3T3-L1 preadipocytes induces differentiation into adipocytes, while expression of the C/EBPδ gene accelerates preadipocyte differentiation. If both genes for C/EBPβ or C/EBPδ are disrupted in 3T3-L1 cells, there is a severe reduction in adipose tissue differentiation. In mice in which the C/EBPβ or C/EBPδ gene is disrupted, white adipose tissue is present at normal levels, but lipid accumulation and UCP-1 in brown adipose tissue is reduced. When both C/EBPβ and C/EBPδ genes are disrupted in mice, most of the animals die of unknown causes in the perinatal period. Of the 15% that survive, there is an extreme reduction in brown adipose tissue and a lesser reduction in white adipose tissue. These observations suggest that C/EBPβ and C/EBPδ play relatively modest roles in white adipocyte differentiation but are important in the development of brown adipose tissue and lipid accumulation.

C/EBPα, along with PPARγ, plays a major role in the induction of preadipocyte differentiation. C/EBPα is expressed at the same time as PPARγ, initiated near the end of the mitotic phase of the 3T3-L1 differentiation programme, just before the expression of adipose-specific genes. Transfection of preadipocytes with the C/EBPα gene blocks mitosis, and the inhibition of the actions of C/EBPα with antisense RNA inhibits differentiation of preadipocytes. These observations suggest that the expression of C/EBPα terminates the clonal expansion of preadipocytes and induces differentiation. When C/EPBα is expressed at the end of the mitotic period of clonal expansion, adipocyte-specific gene expression is initiated, even in the absence of hormonal inducers. Co-expression of C/EBPα and PPARγ in fibroblasts enhances adipocyte formation while co-expression in myoblasts provides a signal strong enough to transform the myoblasts into adipocytes. C/EBPα expression is induced by PPARγ, while C/EBPα reciprocally induces PPARγ expression. C/EBPα and PPARγ act synergistically to induce adipocyte differentiation. In addition, C/EBPα gene expression is autoregulated by the C/EBPα protein. This occurs via interaction with C/EBP response elements in the promoter region of the C/EBPα gene. The primary function of C/EBPα is believed to be maintenance of the differentiated state of adipocytes.

ADD1/SREBP1

The ADD1/SREBP1 transcription factor plays a dual role in adipocyte metabolism. It stimulates adipocyte differentiation and is a key factor in the cholesterol-regulated activation of the transcription of adipocyte-specific lipogenic genes. The cumbersome dual nomenclature for this molecule is due to the independent characterization of ADD1 in rodents and SREBP1 in humans, but its use conveys the dual function of ADD1/SREBP1 in adipocyte differentiation and lipid metabolism. ADD1/SREBP1 belongs to the bHLH family of transcription factors that includes the myogenic regulatory factors that mediate muscle development. ADD1/SREBP1 is stored within the cell as an inactive molecule bound to the membranes of the endoplasmic reticulum. Upon activation, ADD1/SREBP1 is proteolytically cleaved and released from the endoplasmic reticulum. The activated molecule binds to two different sites in the promoter regions of target genes: sterol response elements (SRE) and the typical bHLH sites, the E-box motifs. This dual specificity accounts for the effects of ADD1/SREBP1 on lipid metabolism and adipocyte differentiation.

The presence of ADD1/SREBP1 is required for adipocyte differentiation. However, in contrast to PPARγ, ADD1/SREBP1 alone cannot induce the entire adipogenic programme. When the gene for SREBP1 is disrupted in mice, most of the animals die before parturition. Surviving animals have normal fat levels. Overexpression of ADD1/SREBP1 in pluripotent fibroblasts induces some fibroblasts to differentiate into adipocytes, but only under conditions that are strongly permissive for differentiation, such as the presence of the hormone cocktail used to stimulate adipocyte formation. In the presence of hormonal inducers of differentiation, overexpression of the ADD1/SREBP1 gene in 3T3-L1 preadipocytes increases adipocyte differentiation markers and lipid accumulation compared to hormone treatment alone.

The expression of ADD1/SREBP1 is induced in 3T3-L1 preadipocytes about 12 h after addition of the hormone cocktail that stimulates the differentiation programme. Its expression continues throughout clonal expansion, growth arrest and terminal differentiation of the adipocytes. The timing of ADD1/SREBP expression precedes and overlaps that of PPARγ expression. Thus, ADD1/SREBP1 may induce PPARγ expression and, as ADD1/SREBP1 and PPARγ genes are co-expressed, their actions appear to be synergistic. This synergism is seen in 3T3-L1 preadipocytes transfected with the ADD1/SREBP1 and PPARγ genes. When both genes are present, there is an increase in the adipocyte-specific transcriptional activity over that seen in cells singly transfected with only the ADD1/SREBP1 or PPARγ gene. This synergistic effect is due to ADD1/SREBP1 effects on PPARγ activity. ADD1/SREBP1 is believed to enhance the activity of PPARγ by two separate mechanisms. First, the lipogenic effects of ADD1/SREBP1 may stimulate the synthesis of natural ligands that activate PPARγ. Secondly, ADD1/SREBP1 may directly activate transcription of the PPARγ gene.

In addition to its role in adipogenesis, ADD1/SREBP1 regulates genes for fatty acid, triglycerol and cholesterol metabolism. Enhanced expression of ADD1/SREBP1 is associated with induction of genes associated with increased lipid and cholesterol metabolism, such as glycerol phosphate acyltransferase, LPL and FAS genes. The expression of this transcription factor is regulated by nutrients in mature animals. Under conditions in which lipogenesis is stimulated, as in refeeding after a fasting period, ADD1/SREBP1 expression is increased. Insulin is a potent regulator of ADD1/SREBP1 in adipose tissue and the liver. The elevated levels of insulin that follow nutrient ingestion mediate the effects of nutrient induction of ADD1/SREBP1 expression. Conversely, ADD1/SREBP1 expression is reduced during fasting. A summary of the relationships between the transcription factors that regulate adipogenesis is presented in Fig. 8.3.

Nuclear co-activators and co-repressors: fine-tuning the adipogenic response

The effects of transcription factors on gene transcription are regulated by other nuclear factors called co-activators and co-repressors of transcription. Co-activators of PPARγ and the C/EBPs bind to these transcription factors and enable the maximum activation of gene transcription. The interaction of multiple co-activators with the primary transcription factors at different times adds an additional level and a 'fine-tuning' of the regulation of adipocyte gene transcription. Co-activators of gene expression enhance gene transcription by altering chromosomal chromatin proteins, exposing gene transcription sites on DNA that are usually covered by tightly bound histones and other proteins. Nuclear co-activators also recruit components of the transcriptional apparatus to the gene transcription site.

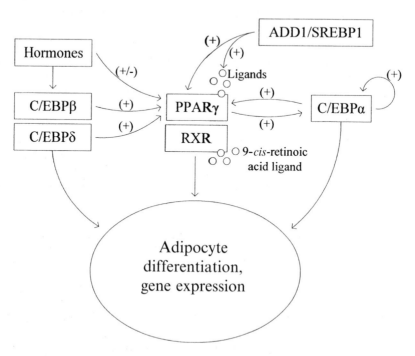

Fig. 8.3. Interrelationships and regulation of adipocyte transcription factors.

Co-activators of PPARγ bind to the carboxyl terminus of these nuclear hormone receptors in the presence of ligand. A complex of co-activators, p160/CBP/p300, bind to PPARγ and attract other activating molecules. The p160/CBP/p300 complex has histone acetyltransferase (HAT) activity. The HAT activity enzymatically acetylates histone protein in chromatin, inducing conformational changes and opening specific gene sites for efficient transcription. The second class of ligand-dependent co-activators is the DRIP/TRAP/ARC complex. Important isoforms of this complex, the proteins DRIP205 and TRAP220, are vital regulatory molecules that share amino acid homologies with a PPARγ-binding protein (PBP).

PPARγ co-activator-1 (PGC-1) is a ligand-independent co-activator of PPARγ that has no HAT activity. Instead, PGC-1 interacts with the p160/CBP/p300 complex that provides HAT activity. PGC-1 is restricted to brown adipose tissue, where its expression is induced by cold stress and alterations in nutrient intake. In brown adipose tissue, PGC-1 stimulates mitochondrial biogenesis and the expression of UCP-1 and components of the cytochrome chain. PGC-2 is also a ligand-independent co-activator of PPARγ. Like PGC-1, PGC-2 has no HAT activity, but may recruit other co-activators with HAT activity to the PPARγ complex.

C/EBPβ interacts with two types of nuclear co-activators. The SWI/SNF complex induces chromatin remodelling in certain cells. As we have seen, the CBP/p300 complex is a strong activator of PPARγ. This complex also activates C/EBPβ. This cross-reactivity of CBP/p300 with PPARγ and C/EBPβ may, in part, explain the synergistic relationship between these two transcription factors in the induction of adipocyte differentiation.

Co-repressors of transcription factors usually bind to the unliganded nuclear receptor and are released upon ligand binding to the receptor. A co-repressor of PPARγ, called Sirt 1 (sirtuin 1), binds to and represses genes activated by PPARγ. Sirt 1 is the mammalian homologue of a molecule that has deacetylase activity. Deacetylase activity may reverse histone acetylation catalysed by co-activators, returning histones to their original binding sites on specific genes and inhibiting gene transcription. Overexpression of the Sirt 1 gene is 3T3-L1 cells interferes with adipogenesis and antisense RNA inhibition of Sirt 1 enhances adipogenesis. In differentiated adipocytes, upregulation of Sirt 1 stimulates lipolysis and reduces fat content.

Hormones and Growth Factors Affecting Preadipocytes and Adipocytes

Insulin

Insulin plays an essential role in stimulating both proliferation and differentiation of preadipocytes. In addition, insulin is a major endocrine regulator of lipogenesis and the maintenance of the differentiated state of mature adipocytes. The main effects of insulin on preadipocytes are to stimulate

differentiation of these cells into adipocytes. Inclusion of IGF-I or pharmacological levels of insulin in the hormone cocktail used to stimulate differentiation of 3T3-L1 cells is required for preadipocyte differentiation. In primary
cell cultures of preadipocytes derived from the stromovascular fraction of
adipose tissue, the inclusion of insulin at physiological levels enhances morphological differentiation and the expression of lipogenic enzymes and their
mRNAs. The presence of glucocorticoids, usually in the form of dexamethasone, and GH enhance insulin action on adipocyte differentiation. On the
other hand, pharmacological levels of insulin (10 µg/ml) induce mitosis in
preadipocytes. This effect is likely mediated by cross-reaction of insulin with
the IGF-I receptor or induction of IGF-I synthesis and secretion by
adipocytes.

In the mature adipocyte and adipose tissue, insulin acts as a lipogenic
hormone, increasing energy storage in the form of triglycerol. Insulin
induces the expression of several lipogenic enzymes, including LPL, FAS
and acetyl-coenzyme A carboxylase. The receptor-mediated effects of
insulin on lipogenic enzymes are mediated by increased expression of the
transcription factors, ADD1/SREBP1, which, in turn, induces PPARγ
expression.

GH and the IGFs

The effects of GH on preadipocytes have been studied extensively. While the
GH receptor is present in preadipocytes and adipocytes, the effects of GH on
adipocyte metabolism, when studied *in vitro*, are variable and hard to reproduce. Some of the conflicting results are due to the differences in metabolism
between cell lines and primary cultures of preadipocytes. When primary cultures of preadipocytes are studied, they are isolated from adipose tissue
using proteolytic enzymes. Exposure of the cells to these enzymes may alter
surface-bound GH receptor concentration or function. This may explain the
differential effects of GH seen in freshly isolated vs longer-term incubations.
GH effects also depend upon the species or cell lines used. This is especially
important when one wishes to study farm animal adipocyte growth and differentiation, as primary cell cultures must be used. There are few or no cell
lines available for domestic animal studies. In addition, GH effects can vary
according to the depot source of fat studied. Different depot sites of adipose
tissue display different metabolism and responses to external factors. All GH
effects require serum at low levels *in vitro*, suggesting that other serum-
borne factors provide a synergistic factor to allow the GH to have an effect
on these cells.

Many studies with GH use preadipocyte cell lines and the results in
these cells often do not coincide with studies in primary cultures of cells
derived from the stromovascular fraction. For example, treatment of
preadipocytes in primary culture with GH does not induce differentiation.
In preadipocyte cell lines, such as the 3T3-L1 and 3T3-F442A cells, however,
physiological levels of GH promote differentiation into adipocytes. GH stimu-

lates proliferation of primary cultures of stromovascular cells, but inhibits proliferation of 3T3-F442A cells. These stimulatory effects of GH on proliferation and differentiation on cells in primary culture are probably mediated by IGF-I. When primary preadipocytes are treated with GH, IGF-I synthesis and secretion are induced. If the effects of IGF-I are inhibited by neutralization with antibodies to IGF-I, proliferation and differentiation are blocked. This provides strong evidence that the effects of GH on preadipocyte proliferation and differentiation are mediated by IGF-I in an autocrine or paracrine manner.

In mature adipocytes treated with GH *in vitro*, GH has differential acute and chronic effects on lipid metabolism. Acute effects are seen in adipose tissue that has been deprived of GH for several hours. These effects are seen in hypophysectomized animals and in cell cultures. Acute exposure of cells to GH induces transient insulin-like, anabolic effects on lipid metabolism, including increased glucose transport and oxidation, increased lipogenesis and reduced lipolysis. After prolonged (1–2 h) exposure of GH *in vitro*, typical GH effects are seen and lipogenesis is reduced. Often, GH induces lipolysis *in vitro*. As discussed in Chapter 5, GH treatment of animals *in vivo* induces lipolysis only under conditions of energy restriction. The reduction in fat mass induced by GH treatment is due to an inhibition of lipogenesis, not the stimulation of lipolysis, when an adequate diet is available. The frequent observation that GH is lipolytic *in vitro* suggests that the cells are in an inadequate nutritional state that allows GH to induce lipolysis. The inhibition of lipogenesis by GH is reflected by the effect of GH on lipogenic enzymes. GH treatment reduces the activity of both FAS and LPL and antagonizes the insulin induction of FAS expression.

Adipocytes and preadipocytes synthesize and secrete IGFs and their binding proteins. In rats, the synthesis of IGFBP-2 and -3 is restricted to preadipocytes, while IGFBP-5 is secreted by both preadipocytes and mature adipocytes. GH regulates the synthesis of IGF-I in adipose tissue. Adipose IGF-I mRNA is stimulated by GH treatment *in vivo* and by GH treatment of preadipocytes *in vitro*. Hypophysectomy of rodents suppresses adipose tissue IGF-I mRNA. The genes for the IGFs are expressed at low levels in preadipocytes *in vitro* and their expression increases during differentiation into mature adipocytes. In stromovascular cell preparations, IGF-I enhances both proliferation and differentiation of preadipocytes. This is reflected by increased expression of enzyme markers of adipocyte differentiation such as α-GPDH and LPL. Low levels of insulin and glucocorticoids act synergistically to enhance the effects of IGF-I on differentiation. IGF-I in serum-free media induces differentiation in 3T3-L1 and primary cultured preadipocytes of most species studied.

In mature adipocytes studied *in vitro*, IGF-I has insulin-like effects. IGF-I treatment increases lipogenesis, glucose uptake and oxidation, and the synthesis and secretion of LPL. As high doses of IGF-I are required for these responses, these effects of IGF-I are thought to be mediated by IGF-I interactions with the insulin receptor. *In vivo* treatment of animals with IGF-I results in a slight or no increase in body fat.

Glucocorticoids

Glucocorticoids are major permissive hormones that are required for the optimal physiological processes of most cells and tissues. The most revealing effects of glucocorticoids on adipose tissue are seen in the clinical syndrome known as Cushing's disease. In individuals with this syndrome, excessive ACTH secretion stimulates excess adrenal glucocorticoid release and elevates circulating glucocorticoid concentrations. A typical phenotype associated with Cushing's disease is the accumulation of large amounts of fat. This suggests that glucocorticoids, at least in the intact animal, stimulate accumulation of lipid stores. When examined *in vitro*, pharmacological levels (0.25–1.0 μM) of glucocorticoids induce differentiation of preadipocytes, but only in the presence of insulin and/or serum. It is not clear whether glucocorticoids are required for, or simply act synergistically with other factors to accelerate adipocyte differentiation. Glucocorticoid effects on adipogenesis are dependent upon the species and cell type, whether primary cells or cell lines, studied. Glucocorticoids stimulate arachidonic acid metabolism to produce the prostaglandin, prostacyclin (PGI_2), and also increase cellular cAMP concentrations. Both are factors that induce adipocyte differentiation.

In mature adipocytes, glucocorticoids play a key role in the regulation of carbohydrate and lipid metabolism. Dexamethasone modulates the expression of many genes involved in adipocyte energy metabolism, including the repression of genes for the IRS-1, the β-adrenergic receptor and the glucose transport protein. Dexamethasone induces the expression of genes for adipsin, LPL, GDPH, phosphoenolpyruvate carboxykinase and pyruvate kinase. These effects are mediated by the nuclear hormone glucocorticoid receptor and which binds to GREs on specific target genes. In differentiated 3T3-L1 cells and adipose tissue, the effects of glucocorticoids are mediated by the activation of C/EBPδ and the repression of C/EBPα transcription. The effects of glucocorticoids act in synergy with C/EBPβ.

Prostaglandins and cAMP

Prostaglandins (PG) are lipid-derived, arachidonic acid derivatives produced by preadipocytes and adipocytes. The major prostaglandin in these cells is prostacyclin (PGI_2). Prostacyclin induces preadipocyte differentiation and activates all PPAR (α, δ, γ) transcription factors. The release of prostacyclin by adipocytes from the OB 1771 cell line can induce differentiation of preadipocytes. Prostacyclin is believed to be the factor that induces adult adipose hyperplasia and differentiation in response to the maturation of fat cells. Another prostaglandin, $PGF_{2\alpha}$ inhibits adipocyte differentiation at physiological concentrations (3×10^{-8} M). $PGF_{2\alpha}$ also induces TGF-α expression in preadipocytes and adipocytes. Other prostaglandins, PGD_2 and 15-deoxy-PGJ_2 may be natural PPARγ ligands, activating PPARγ and inducing differentiation.

cAMP, in general, enhances differentiation of preadipocytes. As discussed in the earlier section on preadipocyte differentiation *in vitro*, the chemical IBMX inhibits phosphodiesterase-catalysed cAMP breakdown. This elevates intracellular cAMP levels and induces preadipocyte differentiation. cAMP-mediated differentiation is accompanied by an induction of the C/EBPβ and PPARγ transcription factors. Treatment of 3T3-L1 cells with prostaglandins also induces cAMP accumulation. As with the effects of prostaglandins on preadipocytes, the effects of cAMP on preadipocytes may depend upon the stage of differentiation, inducing differentiation in early stages and inhibiting it later.

Negative Regulators of Adipose Differentiation

There are several factors that act to oppose the stimulatory effects of hormones and growth factors on the differentiation of adipose tissue. EGF is a 6 kDa single-chain peptide initially discovered in mouse submaxillary salivary glands. It is also present in saliva, blood and urine. EGF promotes the proliferation and differentiation of many mesenchymal and epithelial cell types. EGF acts as a local growth factor in many tissues, including adipose tissue. In preadipocytes, EGF stimulates proliferation and inhibits differentiation at very small, physiological doses (0.6 ng/ml is the 50% effective dose). Treatment of newborn mice for 9 days with EGF decreases body weight, fat mass and the proportion of mature adipocytes in fat depots, by delaying adipocyte differentiation. TGF-α has a significant amino acid sequence homology with EGF and acts via EGF receptor. It is produced by both preadipocytes and adipocytes. Transgenic TGF-α mice display a 40–80% decrease in fat pad weight with an overall decrease of 50% in total body fat. Other potent mitogens such as FGF and PDGF increase preadipocyte proliferation and may inhibit differentiation, although the effects are variable and species-dependent.

TGF-β is a potent inhibitor of adipocyte differentiation. The TGF-β mRNA is present in proliferating preadipocytes and differentiated adipocytes. TGF-β increases the synthesis of the ECM surrounding the adipocytes, and this is believed to inhibit the differentiation of fat cells.

Retinoic acid, a vitamin A metabolite, is a potent inhibitor of adipocyte differentiation in preadipocyte cell lines and primary cultures. All *trans*-retinoic acid binds to the RAR nuclear hormone receptor, which forms dimers with the RXR receptor, the receptor for 9-*cis*-retinoic acid. Retinoic acid and PPARγ competition for limited RXR may inhibit the stimulatory effects of PPARγ on differentiation (recall that PPARγ forms dimers with RXR). Alternatively, the RAR/RXR complex acts as a retinoic acid-dependent activator or repressor of gene transcription. Retinoic acid acts very early in the adipocyte differentiation programme, immediately after the hormonal induction of differentiation, but before the expression of C/EBPα. Retinoic acid acts to inhibit the expression of C/EBPα and PPARγ, but has no effect on C/EBPβ expression.

Adipose tissue as an endocrine organ

Adipose tissue is not simply a static reservoir for lipid deposition and mobilization. It has recently been shown that adipocytes secrete a variety of local and systemic factors which regulate appetite, energy homeostasis, the immune response and vascular development. The newly discovered endocrine properties of adipose tissue expand the functional role of this seemingly innocuous tissue to that of a regulatory entity. New information about the regulatory role of adipose tissue, at both the local and systemic levels, has led to a reassessment of the function of this tissue and the factors that regulate metabolism and growth. In the future, this new functional role of adipose tissue may lead to new methods for the regulation of animal production. Some of the factors secreted by adipocytes and their regulatory functions are discussed in this section.

Leptin will be discussed fully in Chapter 11. Leptin is a prominent secreted hormone of adipose tissue that acts in a classical endocrine manner. It was the first adipose tissue hormone identified when it was discovered in 1994. Initially, there was a great deal of anticipation that this adipocyte-derived, appetite-suppressing, fat-reducing hormone would provide an effective treatment for human obesity. Unfortunately, this has not proven to be the case. Nevertheless, leptin remains an important hormone that regulates appetite, energy storage and fertility. A more complete understanding of its effects may yet provide another means to regulate appetite, carcass composition and animal production efficiency. Manipulation of its actions on the reproductive system has the potential to provide major alterations in the reproductive efficiency of farm animals.

Adiponectin is the most abundant gene product of human adipose tissue. It occurs at very high levels in plasma (5–30 µg/ml). Adiponectin is also called adipocyte complement-related protein of 30 kDa (Acrp30) and AdipoQ. Adiponectin shares homologies with the immune protein complement Clq and is thought to play a role in the inhibition of inflammatory pathways. Adiponectin also has metabolic effects on lipid and carbohydrate in liver, skeletal muscle and adipose tissue. Adiponectin enhances insulin sensitivity in the liver, reducing hepatic glucose output in response to insulin. The secretion of adiponectin is induced by IGF-I, insulin and PPARγ ligands, such as the TZDs. Its expression is suppressed by treatment with β-agonists and glucocorticoids.

TNF-α is a 17 kDa polypeptide that is named for its ability to induce tumour necrosis when injected into tumours *in vivo*. Many tissues produce TNF-α, including skeletal muscle, lymphoid tissue and the adipocytes in adipose tissue. While TNF-α is found in the circulation, it likely acts locally in adipose tissue by autocrine and paracrine mechanisms. This growth factor inhibits differentiation of preadipocytes into adipocytes *in vitro*. On the other hand, TNF-α can induce dedifferentiation of mature adipocytes, acting by a reduction of PPARγ and C/EBPα expression. TNF-α induces preadipocyte and adipocyte apoptosis and induces lipolysis of fat stores *in vivo* and *in vitro*. These observations suggest that TNF-α may function to limit adipose tissue mass in the animal.

Resistin is a 10 kDa polypeptide that is produced solely by adipose tissue. Its name is derived from early observations that resistin conferred insulin resistance on obese rodents. It has since been shown that resistin is not related to human insulin resistance. Resistin expression is increased during differentiation, by feeding, obesity and insulin. Resistin acts by endocrine, autocrine and paracrine pathways to inhibit adipocyte differentiation, possibly via a feedback mechanism that restricts adipocyte formation. Resistin expression is suppressed by fasting, diabetes and PPARγ agonists, such as the TZDs. Its physiological role in the adult is still unknown.

The renin–angiotensin system is an osmoregulatory system that modulates fluid balance and vascular tone, playing an important role in the regulation of blood pressure. The components of the classical system are secreted by the kidneys and liver and are found in the circulation. Renin, secreted by the kidneys, is a proteolytic enzyme that cleaves hepatic-derived angiotensinogen to angiotensin I, which is converted to the active octapeptide, angiotensin II. Adipose tissue also synthesizes all components of this system and it is believed that the adipose-derived angiotensin II acts locally by autocrine and paracrine mechanisms. Adipose tissue also contains receptors for angiotensin II. Local angiotensin II regulates adipose tissue blood supply by stimulating angiogenesis during adipogenesis. Angiotensin II also stimulates preadipocyte differentiation into adipocytes. This is mediated by the stimulation of PGI_2 synthesis. Angiotensin II stimulates lipogenesis in mature adipocytes. Adipose tissue angiotensinogen production is upregulated by nutrients. This observation, as well as the effects of angiotensin II on lipid metabolism, suggests that angiotensin may play a role in the regulation of body weight and body composition.

Further Reading

Ailhaud, G., Grimaldi, P. and Negrel, R. (1992) Cellular and molecular aspects of adipose tissue development. *Annual Review of Nutrition* 12, 207–233.

Butterwith, S.C. (1994) Molecular events in adipocyte development. *Pharmacology and Therapeutics* 61, 399–411.

Ferre, P. (2004) The biology of peroxisome proliferator-activated receptors; relationship with lipid metabolism and insulin sensitivity. *Diabetes* 53(Suppl. 1), S43–S50.

Gregoire, F.M. (2001) Adipocyte differentiation: from fibroblast to endocrine cell. *Experimental Biology and Medicine* 226, 997–1002.

Gregoire, F.M., Smas, C.M. and Sul, H.S. (1998) Understanding adipocyte differentiation. *Physiological Reviews* 78, 783–809.

Hausman, G.J. (1989) The influence of insulin, triiodothyronine (T_3) and insulin-like growth factor-I (IGF-I) on the differentiation of preadipocytes in serum-free cultures of pig stromal-vascular cells. *Journal of Animal Science* 67, 3136–3143.

Hausman, G.J., Jewell, D.E. and Hentges, E.J. (1989) Endocrine regulation of adipogenesis. In: Campion, D.R., Hausman, G.J. and Martin, R.J. (eds) *Animal Growth Regulation*. Plenum Press, New York, pp. 49–68.

Kim, S. and Moustaid-Moussa, N. (2000) Secretory, endocrine and autocrine/paracrine function of the adipocyte. *Journal of Nutrition* 130, 3110S–3115S.

Lazar, M.A. (1999) PPARγ in adipocyte differentiation. *Journal of Animal Science* 77(Suppl. 3), 16–22.

Louveau, I. and Gondret, F. (2004) Regulation of development and metabolism of adipose tissue by growth hormone and the insulin-like growth factor system. *Domestic Animal Endocrinology* 27, 241–255.

Mondrup, S. and Lane, M.D. (1997) Regulating adipogenesis. *The Journal of Biological Chemistry* 272, 5367–5370.

Nawrocki, A.R. and Scherer, P.E. (2004) The delicate balance between fat and muscle: adipokines in metabolic disease and musculoskeletal inflammation. *Current Opinion in Pharmacology* 4, 281–289.

Ntambi, J.M. and Kim, Y.-C. (2000) Adipocyte differentiation and gene expression. *Journal of Nutrition* 130, 3122S–3126S.

Picard, F., Kurtev, M., Chung, N., Topark-Ngarm, A., Senawong, T., de Oliveira, R.M., Leid, M., McBurney, M.W. and Guarente, L. (2004) Sirt1 promotes fat mobilization in white adipocytes by repressing PPAR-γ. *Nature* 429, 771–776.

Prins, J.B. (2002) Adipose tissue as an endocrine organ. *Best Practice and Research. Clinical Endocrinology and Metabolism* 16, 639–651.

Rebuffe-Scrive, M., Krotkiewski, M., Elfverson, J. and Bjorntorp, P. (1988) Muscle and adipose tissue morphology and metabolism in Cushing's syndrome. *Journal of Clinical Endocrinology and Metabolism* 67, 1122–1128.

Rosen, E.D., Walkey, C.J., Puigserver, P. and Spiegelman, B.M. (2004) Transcriptional regulation of adipogenesis. *Genes and Development* 14, 1239–1307.

Serrero, G. and Lepak, N. (1996) Endocrine and paracrine negative regulators of adipose differentiation. *International Journal of Obesity* 20(Suppl. 3), S58–S64.

9   Steroids and Animal Growth

Steroids are complex, water-insoluble, lipid-like compounds which are synthesized from cholesterol. Ruminants are unique in that they are the only animals which have a positive growth response to oestrogens, the female steroid hormones. Oestrogens were the first growth promotants to be studied and used to enhance production efficiency in farm animals. In ruminants, oestrogens increase muscle growth and fat deposition of castrated males. As they are relatively abundant, cheap and provide reliable responses to enhance growth and alter body composition, they are still widely used in animal production.

Types, sources and functions of the major naturally occurring steroids are shown in Table 9.1. Steroids can be divided into two broad categories, based upon their source and function: the first are the so-called sex steroids, produced by the gonads (ovaries, testes) and the placenta, and, second, the adrenal steroids. Glucocorticoids, also called corticosteroids and corticoids, such as cortisol and corticosterone, are products of the adrenal cortex, the outer portion of the adrenal gland. Physiologically, the adrenocortical steroids are involved primarily in the mobilization of carbohydrates and amino acids in response to food deprivation or stress. The function of these hormones has been discussed in previous chapters. The focus of the current chapter is on the sex steroids and their effects on farm animal growth.

The naturally occurring female sex steroids, produced by the ovaries, include oestrogens, the most potent of which is oestradiol-17β. Oestrogens function to regulate reproduction and are responsible for the secondary sexual characteristics of females, such as maintenance of the uterus and mammary glands, distribution and quantity of fat and muscle, and, in humans, smooth skin, small larynx and lack of facial hair. Diethylstilbestrol (DES) is a potent synthetic, non-steroidal oestrogen first synthesized in 1938. In the late 1940s, it was shown to increase ADG in heifers, sheep and poultry. It was patented in the early 1950s by Wise Burroughs as stilbestrol and was the impetus for the formation of Elanco by the Eli Lily Corporation in 1954. DES is no longer in use. It was banned in 1979, as a potential carcinogen. Other oestrogens which are still widely used in ruminant animal growth stimulation include oestradiol-17β, oestradiol benzoate, zeranol, dienestrol and

Table 9.1. General characteristics of steroids.

Steroid type	Examples	Source	Function
Oestrogen	Oestradiol-17β	Ovary	Reproduction, 2° sexual characteristics
Progestins	Progesterone	Ovary, placenta	Reproduction, 2° sexual characteristics
Androgens	Testosterone	Testis	Reproduction, 2° sexual characteristics
Corticosteroids (glucocorticoids)	Cortisol, corticosterone	Adrenal cortex	Carbohydrate metabolism

Hexestrol®. The structures for oestrogens, progestins and androgens are shown in Fig. 9.1.

Progestins are the second major family of naturally occurring sex steroids in females. Progesterone is the naturally occurring progestin in females. Progesterone has direct effects on the uterus, priming it for pregnancy by stimulating its growth and differentiation. Progesterone is also responsible for the maintenance of pregnancy in mammals. Naturally occurring progesterone is secreted by the corpus luteum of the ovary after ovulation and is elevated during the latter part of the oestrous cycle. If conception and pregnancy occur, progesterone levels remain elevated, and along with oestrogen, progesterone prepares the uterus to receive the embryo and maintain pregnancy. Removal of progesterone results in the immediate termination of pregnancy.

Progestins, such as the naturally occurring progesterone and potent synthetics like melengestrol acetate (MGA), enhance growth and feed efficiency

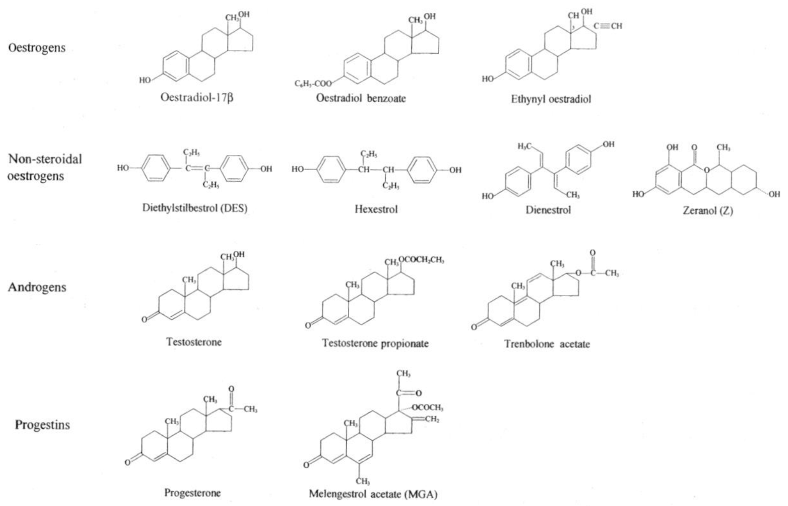

Fig. 9.1. Chemical structures of oestrogens, androgens and progestins.

(FE) in cyclic heifers. This is thought to be primarily an effect on behaviour, although there is some evidence that progesterone increases the half-life of oestrogens when given in combination. The natural role of progesterone involves not only effects on the uterus, but also includes behavioural effects on the mother, inducing a relatively calm state, which is conducive to pregnancy. Oestrogens have the opposite effect, inducing erratic, frenzied behaviour in females during the heat phase of the oestrous cycle. The word 'oestrus' is derived from the Greek for 'gadfly', a term suggesting the erratic behaviour seen in animals in heat. The positive effects of progestins in enhancing farm animal growth are thought to be a result of the 'calming' effect of progestins in female animals. This counteracts the hyperactivity induced by oestrogen and allows energy to be directed to body growth as opposed to energy use in oestrogen-induced hyperactivity.

The androgen steroids are produced by the testis of the male and are the predominant steroids in the male. Testosterone is the primary circulating natural androgen produced by the testes. Testosterone is converted to its active metabolite, dihydrotestosterone (DHT), in most target tissues by the enzyme 5α-reductase. Androgens are responsible for the typical male secondary sexual characteristics, such as maintenance of the accessory sex glands (prostate, seminal vesicles, bulbourethral gland) that produce seminal fluids, the external male genitalia and sperm production by the testis. They also have distinct effects on the CNS. These effects are manifested in the induction of the sex drive, or libido, in both sexes, as well as aggressive nature of male animals to maintain dominance during the mating season. In humans, androgens induce laryngeal growth, beard growth and hair loss. Aside from the reproductive system, one of the primary target tissues for androgens is skeletal muscle. The anabolic effects of androgens on male skeletal muscle are responsible for the typical sexual dimorphism of mammals. In most species, males are larger, with a greater proportion of muscle than females.

Another important function of the sex steroids includes effects on bone growth and maturation. In the pre-pubertal animal, low doses of the sex steroids increase linear bone growth and bone mass. The growth spurt at puberty is largely the result of maturation of the gonads and the outpouring of androgens in males and oestrogens in females. Later on, when growth ceases, higher circulating levels of oestrogens and androgens stimulate the epiphyseal growth plates to undergo fusion or closure as they transform from cartilaginous structures into mature bone.

Several commercial formulations of anabolic steroids have been approved by the Food and Drug Administration (FDA) as livestock production enhancers in the USA. The trade names, formulations and their target animals are provided in Table 9.2.

Oestrogens and Ruminant Growth

It has long been known that castrated males have more fat tissue and less lean tissue than non-castrated males. Thus, these animals have a lower FE

Table 9.2. Anabolic steroid formulations and their uses in farm animals.

Trade name	Composition	For use in
Synovex-S	20 mg Oestradiol benzoate and 200 mg progesterone	Steers
Synovex-H	20 mg Oestradiol benzoate and 200 mg testosterone propionate	Heifers
Ralgro	36 mg Zeranol	Steers
		Heifers
		Calves
	12 mg Zeranol	Lambs
MGA	Melengestrol acetate 0.25–0.50 mg/day	Heifers
Compudose	24 mg Oestradiol-17β	Steers
		Heifers
		Calves
Steer-oid	20 mg Oestradiol benzoate and 200 mg progesterone	Steers
Synovex-C	10 mg Oestradiol-17β and 100 mg progesterone	Calves
Heifer-oid	20 mg Oestradiol benzoate and 200 mg testosterone propionate	Heifers
Finaplix-S	140 mg Trenbolone acetate	Steers
Finaplix-H	200 mg Trenbolone acetate	Heifers
Revalor-S	120 mg Trenbolone acetate and 24 mg oestradiol-17β	Steers
Revalor-H	140 mg Trenbolone acetate and 14 mg oestradiol-17β	Heifers

than intact males. Oestrogen treatment of castrated male ruminants such as wethers and steers increases ADG and FE by 10% to 20%, with only a small increase in feed intake (FI). Along with these production effects there is an increase in lean tissue deposition (including bone and connective tissue), bone density and protein and water deposition. At the same time, subcutaneous and intramuscular fat, along with carcass grade, are reduced. Typical effects of oestrogens on performance and carcass characteristics of steers are shown in Table 9.3. These are the results after 164 days of treatment with oestrogen implants. Steers were implanted with Synovex-S or Ralgro on day 1 only (single) or on day 1 and day 70 (reimplanted group). Oestradiol-17β (E_2) was given as a controlled-release silicon rubber implant. No statistical differences were seen between treatments with oestradiol and progesterone or Zeranol or oestradiol-17β. There were no differences in the source of oestrogen on performance characteristics but characteristics were improved by oestrogen treatment over non-treated animals.

When oestrogens are given to intact (non-castrated) ruminant males, only small, variable effects are observed. There is a reduction of aggression in bulls and, in general, there is an increase in body fat in both sheep and cattle. As might be expected, females have a much lower response to exogenous oestrogens, which induce only minor effects.

Oestrogens and Non-ruminants

Oestrogens are less effective as production enhancers in non-ruminants, although they do have effects on production and body composition. For example, in boars, oestrogens increase ADG and per cent body fat, while reducing boar odour (taint) in meat. In addition, oestrogens slightly increase FI, FE and nitrogen retention in boars. In barrows and gilts, there are few if any beneficial effects of oestrogen treatment. In these animals, oestrogen increases udder growth with a concomitant reduction in belly (bacon) value. In poultry, oestrogen treatment increases both subcutaneous and intramuscular body fat by 55%, while FI in increased by about 20%. This results in a reduction of FE by 8%. For these reasons, oestrogens are not used as production enhancers in poultry.

Table 9.3. Effects of oestrogen implants on growth and carcass characteristics of steers.

Treatment	ADG (kg)	%	FI (kg/day)	%	FE	%	Cutability
Control	1.22	–	8.32	–	6.91	–	49.1
Single	1.30	7.1	8.68	4.3	6.74	2.5	49.1
Reimplant	1.40	15.1	8.86	6.5	6.37	7.8	49.1
E_2	1.38	13.2	8.73	4.9	6.39	7.5	49.0

From Basson *et al.* (1985). FE is given as feed consumed per unit gain. Improvement over control animals is shown as %.

Androgens and Ruminant Growth

Androgens, the male reproductive hormones, also are used in regulating farm animal growth. Unlike oestrogens, it is not particularly surprising that androgens might be used as growth enhancers, as their normal physiological role in the male includes the stimulation of skeletal muscle growth. One needs to look only at the larger body, heavy forequarters and relatively lean form of a bull compared to steers or heifers to gain an appreciation for the anabolic effects of androgens on body form and composition. Unfortunately, androgens also have strong behavioural effects, inducing competition for hierarchy and for dominance in mating. This includes, of course, typical male behaviour such as aggressiveness and fighting. While an important part of animal behaviour and successful propagation of the species, these traits are unwanted in animal production systems. Like the gadfly female, the bull-headed and combative male wastes energy (and induces bruises and wounds) with this aggressive behaviour. Hence, farm animal males are traditionally castrated, in part to avoid these behaviours.

Androgens increase ADG and carcass quality in steers, lambs and heifers. Trenbolone acetate (TBA) is a synthetic androgen that has strong anabolic effects on growth, but is only weakly androgenic, eliminating many of the unwanted behavioural traits. It was approved for use in steers and heifers in 1987. Androgens are most effective in castrated males when they are given in combination with oestrogen. This results in an additive response, with improved production efficiency and carcass characteristics over that seen with either steroid given alone (Table 9.4). Compared with oestrogen treatment, TBA is less effective in inducing positive growth performance characteristics, but has more dramatic effects on carcass composition. When given in combination with oestrogen, additive effects are seen, with larger increases in ADG and FE than seen with single steroid treatment.

As with oestrogens, the effects of androgens on animal growth and body composition vary with the species and gender of the animal. In intact males,

Table 9.4. Effects of oestrogen and androgens given alone or in combination on growth and carcass characteristics in steers.

Treatment	ADG (kg)	%	FE	%	Yield grade (YG)	Cutability
Control	1.39	–	6.79	–	2.51	49.96
E_2	1.55	11.5	6.29	7.4	2.43	50.14
TBA	1.49	7.2	6.29	7.4	2.25	50.54
E_2 + TBA	1.62	16.5	5.95	12.4	2.29	50.38

Adapted from Trenkle (1987).

there is an increase in ADG and carcass leanness, with better FE than castrates. Androgen-treated males have larger forequarters, neck and crest than females or castrated males, as these muscles are more androgen-sensitive. In addition, behaviour problems typical of males, such as fighting, are common in androgenized animals. In heifers, TBA increases ADG, nitrogen retention and protein deposition. In beef and dairy cows, TBA increases carcass lean tissue while reducing fat deposition.

Mechanism of Action of Steroids in Ruminant Growth

As noted above, ruminants are unique in their growth response to oestrogens. Oestrogens are female hormones that are primarily involved in the regulation of reproductive events. Compared to males, females are generally smaller-framed animals, with smaller muscle masses and larger proportions of body fat. Human females are characterized by their narrower shoulders, wider hips, breasts and absence of facial hair. Thus, it is a bit of a paradox that oestrogenic hormones would induce ruminant males to grow faster and accumulate lean tissue mass. A lingering mystery in animal biology is 'How do oestrogens induce muscle growth in ruminants?' Several hypotheses have been introduced and examined experimentally.

Of course, the possibility that oestrogens have direct effects on growth is the first that one would propose and examine. If oestrogens are having a direct effect on skeletal muscle, they must act through muscle receptors and one would expect to see either increased numbers of skeletal muscle oestrogen receptors or an increase in the response of ruminant skeletal muscle to the direct effects of oestrogens. Oestrogen receptors are indeed present in ovine and bovine skeletal muscle, but their concentrations are very low, i.e. only 1% of uterine concentrations. In addition, similar levels of the oestrogen receptors are also seen in rat muscle, which does not have a growth response to oestrogen. These observations argue against a direct effect of oestrogens on ruminant skeletal muscle.

Oestrogens may act by indirect mechanisms in the living animal. Oestrogens may act by inducing another hormone, which, in turn, affects the growth of muscle. With the knowledge that GH has significant and strong effects on skeletal muscle growth and development, scientists sought evidence that perhaps circulating GH mediated the effects of oestrogens. This hypothesis was supported by the observations that oestradiol-17β and GH have similar effects on nitrogen balance in ruminants. Both act to conserve body nitrogen stores and increase lean tissue deposition. This is reflected by reduced urinary nitrogen and circulating amino acid concentrations in response to both GH and oestradiol-17β. Evidence was accumulated that GH mediates the effects of oestrogen by demonstrating that oestrogen treatment increases pituitary weight and GH release in animals. In addition, oestrogen treatment of sheep anterior pituitary cells grown *in vitro* induced the release of GH by the cells. Although similar studies using bovine anterior pituitary cells failed to demonstrate this release immediately, pretreatment of the cells with oestradiol-17β sensitized the cells to the action of GHRH that then increased the GH release. This provided tantalizing evidence that perhaps oestrogens were acting via the pituitary/hypothalamic system to stimulate GH release.

Unfortunately, there are problems with this hypothesis. For example, the treatment of animals with both GH and oestradiol-17β results in additive effects. This suggests that these compounds act through independent pathways. Both GH and oestradiol-17β stimulate nitrogen retention in ruminants, as reflected by a reduction of circulating urea nitrogen, amino acids and urinary nitrogen. Oestrogens have effects similar to GH on production characteristics such as ADG and FE, and carcass protein and water as well as bone deposition. In addition, it has been shown that the positive effects of oestrogens on protein deposition may result from an inhibition of protein degradation. GH, on the other hand, has no effect on protein degradation and increases muscle protein accretion by increasing protein synthesis. In laboratory rodents that do not have a growth response to oestrogen, oestrogen also induces an increase in GH. These observations provide evidence that the effects of oestrogen are not mediated by GH, at least in a straightforward manner.

Similarly, an indirect mechanism of oestrogen involving GH might act through the GH receptor. Although GH receptors are present in many tissues, hepatic GH receptors are abundant and mediate the GH induction of IGF-I secretion by the liver. IGF-I, in turn, mediates many of the effects of GH, especially those in skeletal muscle. In steers implanted with oestrogen, liver GH receptors are increased by 250%. This suggests that oestrogen effects may be mediated by an increased hepatic sensitivity to GH, with no or minor increases in circulating GH, resulting in increased circulating IGF-I. Oestrogen implants increase plasma IGF-I levels, and this may provide an explanation for the additive effects of oestrogen and GH, as GH also increases IGF-I concentration in the circulation.

Androgen mechanisms of action

Interestingly, natural and synthetic androgens have different mechanisms of action. Testosterone and DHT increase both muscle protein synthesis and degradation, although the effect on stimulating protein synthesis predominates, resulting in net protein deposition. The synthetic androgen, TBA, on the other hand, reduces both protein degradation and synthesis. As TBA has a greater effect on decreasing protein degradation, there is an overall increase in muscle protein deposition.

Like oestrogens, the mechanism of action of androgens in promoting muscle growth and altering body composition is controversial. Skeletal muscle contains androgen receptors, which bind both testosterone and the TBA metabolite, 17α-methyl-TBA. This provides a pathway for the direct action of androgens on skeletal muscle growth.

In addition, several candidates which may mediate the effects of androgens have been investigated. It has been proposed that these indirect effects of androgens are, in part, due to suppression of the effects of adrenal glucocorticoids. Corticosteroids reduce protein synthesis and stimulate protein degradation, mobilizing amino acids for gluconeogenesis under conditions of stress or food restriction. Treatment with TBA reduces cortisol levels while increasing protein deposition. This suggests that cortisol may play a permissive role in mediating androgen effects and that reduction of endogenous corticosteroid levels by androgens allows the anabolic effects of androgens to be expressed.

Likewise, circulating concentrations of the thyroid hormones, specifically T_4, are reduced by androgen treatment. The natural role of T_4 is to increase energy expenditure in the form of increased oxidative metabolism and muscle protein degradation. Thus, the reduction of T_4 concentrations by androgens may contribute to the enhanced energy efficiency of treated animals, as energy requirements and protein degradation are reduced in the treated animal.

Finally, the effects of androgens on ruminant growth may actually be mediated by oestrogens. Androgens are converted by peripheral tissues, including skeletal muscle, into oestrogens, which may act as a local stimulant for muscle growth. Treatment of animals with TBA implants decreases the clearance rate of oestrogens in steers, heifers and ewes and increases concentrations of circulating oestradiol-17β. All of these processes lead to increased concentrations of oestradiol-17β in the circulation, and to the speculation that, in addition to direct effects of androgens mediated by skeletal muscle receptors, some effects of androgens may be mediated by oestrogens.

Treatment of ruminants with a combination of oestrogens and androgens leads to additive effects in steers, providing optimal growth rates in castrated animals. This combination treatment has no effect on GH concentrations of treated animals, suggesting that effects of combination treatment may be direct, without involvement of the endocrine somatotrophic axis.

In light of our relatively recent knowledge that some hormones, such as IGF-I, can act as both endocrine factors and local growth factors, without the intervention of the circulatory system, re-examination of the interactions of steroids, GH and IGF-I at the local level have provided new insight into the regulation of animal growth by anabolic steroids. In steers treated with Revalor-S (TBA + oestradiol-17β) for 32 to 38 days, IGF-I mRNA levels in liver and semi-membranous muscle were increased by 50% to 70%, while circulating IGF-I was increased by 30% to 40%. In addition, this treatment induced the number of actively proliferating satellite cells isolated from the semi-membranous muscle. This suggests that a combination of oestrogenic and androgenic steroids induced synthesis of IGF-I in skeletal muscle, and the increased local IGF-I activated the normally resting satellite cells in a local autocrine or paracrine manner (White *et al.*, 2003).

References and Further Reading

Basson, R.P., Dinusson, W.E., Embry, L., Feller, D.L., Gorham, P.E., Htiryrt, H.P., Hinman, D.D., McAskill, J., Parrott, C., Riley, J., Stanton, T.L., Young, D.C. and Wagner, J.F. (1985) Comparison of the performance of estradiol silicone rubber implant-treated steers to that of zear-alanol or estradiol + progesterone. *Journal of Animal Science* 61, 1023–1036.

Burroughs, W., Culbertson, C.C., Kastelic, J., Cheng, E. and Hale, W.H. (1954) The effects of trace amounts of diethylstilbe-strol in rations of fattening steers. *Science* 120, 66–68.

Buttery, P.J. and Sinnett-Smith, P.A. (1984) The mode of action of anabolic agents with special reference to their effects on protein metabolism – some speculations. In: Roche, J.F. and O'Callagan, D. (eds) *Manipulation of Growth in Farm Animals.* Martinus Nijhoff, The Hague, The Netherlands, pp. 210–232.

Duckett, S.K. and Andrae, J.G. (2001) Implant strategies in an integrated beef produc-tion system. *Journal of Animal Science* 79(Suppl. E), E110–E117.

Hancock, D.L., Wagner, J.F. and Anderson, D.B. (1991) Effects of estrogens and androgens on animal growth. In: Pearson, A.M. and Dutson, T.R. (eds) *Advances in Meat Science*, Vol. 7. Elsevier Applied Science, New York and London, pp. 255–297.

O'Lamhna, M. and Roche, J.F. (1984) Recent studies with anabolic agents in steers and bulls. In: Roche, J.F. and O'Callaghan, D. (eds) *Manipulation of Growth in Farm Animals.* Martinus Nijhoff, The Hague, The Netherlands, pp. 100–111.

Roche, J.F. and Quirke, J.F. (1986) The effects of steroid hormones and xenobiotics on growth of farm animals. In: Buttrey, P.J., Haynes, N.B. and Lindsay, D.B. (eds) *Control and Manipulation of Animal Growth.* Butterworths, London, pp. 39–51.

Trenkle, A. (1987) Combining TBA, estrogen implants results in additive growth pro-moting effects in steers. *Feedstuffs* 26, 43.

White, M.E., Johnson, B.J., Hathaway, M.R. and Dayton, W.R. (2003) Growth factor messenger RNA levels in muscle and liver of steroid-implanted and nonim-planted steers. *Journal of Animal Science* 81, 965–972.

10 Catecholamines, Beta-agonists and Nutrient Repartitioning

Living organisms are subjected to stress on a daily basis. Animals living in the wild must deal with environmental challenges, such as cold, heat, rain, wind or snow, as well as predator attacks and competition for food, habitat and reproductive partners. Many of these daily stresses have been minimized or eliminated in domestic animals that are provided with food, shelter and protection from predators. Nevertheless, the survival response to daily challenges is an innate characteristic that allows an animal to cope with the daily stresses to which it is subjected. This highly evolved physiological system that ensures an animal will survive stress, prosper and propagate is regulated by components of the CNS, the autonomic nervous system and the endocrine system.

When an animal is challenged by a threat, such as a predator or a mating competitor, it can respond in two ways. It can either defend itself, its mate and offspring, or it can flee for safety, hoping to elude a more powerful foe. This behavioural response to stress was termed the 'fight or flight' syndrome by W.B. Cannon in 1932. This self-preservation response is accompanied by an array of acute physiological adaptations that mobilize energy and provide it to organ systems involved in this reflex. The sympathetic portion of the autonomic nervous system and the adrenal glands are largely responsible for changes in the cardiovascular, respiratory and gastrointestinal systems that mediate the response to stress. These processes are stimulated by the release of catecholamines such as norepinephrine, a neurotransmitter in the SNS, and the adrenal gland hormone epinephrine. This results in the mobilization of lipids and glycogen and their catabolism by lipolysis and glycogenolysis to provide energy to the animal. In addition, coordinated responses in the cardiovascular system occur. The rate and strength of heart contractions are increased and vasoconstriction of blood vessels reduces blood flow to the gastrointestinal tract. Concomitantly, vasodilation of blood vessels increases blood flow to skeletal muscle, the heart and the brain. In total, these physiological adaptations ensure that organs involved in response to 'fight or flight' stress receive the energy needed for optimal function. While one might properly assume that a response to acute stress that involves the mobilization and use of body energy stores is a process that is counter to the use of energy for growth, nevertheless, it has been recently found that catecholamine derivatives are useful as agents to alter food animal body composition and improve production efficiency.

The Autonomic Nervous System and the Adrenal Medulla

The autonomic nervous system is part of the peripheral nervous system that lies outside of, but arises from the CNS. The autonomic nervous system is responsible for the innervation of the skin, visceral organs, blood vessels, smooth muscles and glands of the body and regulates the involuntary reactions that characterize the functions of these tissues. The autonomic nervous system is divided into two portions, the SNS and the parasympathetic nervous system (Fig. 10.1). Parasympathetic neurones originate in the craniosacral regions of the spinal cord, while those of the SNS arise from the

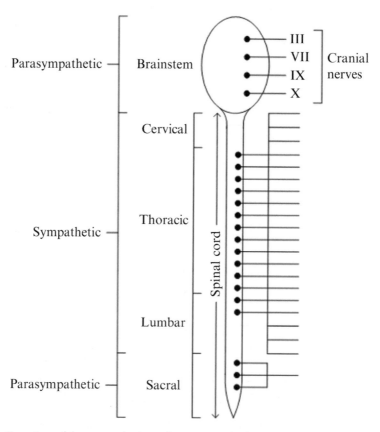

Fig. 10.1. Overview of the sympathetic and parasympathetic nervous systems.

thoracolumbar regions of the spinal cord. In contrast to the somatic nervous system, in which a single continuous nerve fibre extends to innervate muscle, neurones from the autonomic nervous system form synapses once they have left the CNS. After leaving the spinal cord, the preganglionic neurones for the autonomic nervous system terminate in ganglia, clusters of neuronal cell bodies where the synapses occur (Fig. 10.2). The nerve fibres then continue on to their target tissues as postganglionic neurones. Sympathetic ganglia lie close to the spinal cord in a distinct chain of neurones, the sympathetic trunk, or they are located halfway between the spinal cord and the affected organ. In contrast, parasympathetic ganglia are located within the walls of the affected organ, characterized by a short postganglionic fibre. In both pre- and postganglionic parasympathetic neurones acetylcholine acts as the neurotransmitter. On the other hand, the SNS uses acetylcholine as the preganglionic neurotransmitter but the postganglionic neurotransmitter is norepinephrine, a catecholamine.

The adrenal medulla is a specialized modification of the SNS and is part of the sympathoadrenal system. This system includes the SNS and the catecholamine hormone secretions of the adrenal medulla. Like the pituitary gland, the adrenal gland is derived from more than one embryonic source. The outer cortex, source of the glucocorticoids, is of mesodermal origin. The inner medulla, which synthesizes and secretes the catecholamines, is derived from embryonic neural crest cells, which arise near the spinal cord.

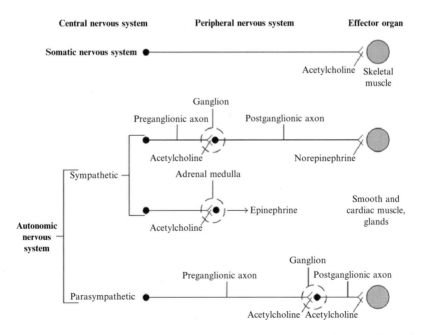

Fig. 10.2. Comparison of the somatic and autonomic nervous systems, their ganglia and neurotransmitters.

The preganglionic neurones that regulate the adrenal medulla arise from the spinal cord and terminate in the adrenal medulla. Unlike other sympathetic nerves, however, there is no postganglionic nerve fibre and the adrenal medulla, instead, secretes its products, the catecholamine hormones, directly into the bloodstream. The primary catecholamine produced and secreted by the adrenal medulla of most mammals is epinephrine, a hormone closely related to norepinephrine, the neurotransmitter of postganglionic sympathetic nerves. Epinephrine is released in response to preganglionic nerve stimulation from the SNS and influences adrenergic receptors throughout the body.

In mammals, the most abundant catecholamines are adrenaline (also called epinephrine), noradrenaline (norepinephrine) and dopamine. The catecholamines are amino acid derivatives that are synthesized from tyrosine (Fig. 10.3). This involves an initial hydroxylation of tyrosine to form dihydroxyphenylalanine (DOPA), followed by a decarboxylation resulting in dopamine formation. Hydroxylation of dopamine produces norepinephrine, which is then methylated to form epinephrine. The presence of the amino methyl group on epinephrine distinguishes it from norepinephrine (the prefix 'nor', means 'without'). As shown in Table 10.1, epinephrine, norepinephrine and dopamine are found in the circulation in very low levels which are quite variable between species. Although norepinephrine and dopamine are found in the circulation, they are primarily neurotransmitters that function within the nervous system. Very high concentrations of norepinephrine are needed to induce a response in endocrine target organs. For example, in humans, norepinephrine concentrations above 1800 pg/ml are needed to

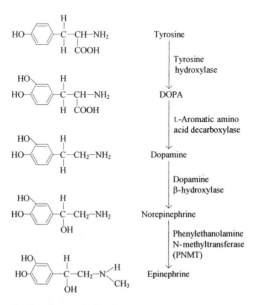

Fig. 10.3. Biological synthesis of catecholamines.

Table 10.1. Plasma concentration (pg/ml) of catecholamines in various species.

Catecholamine	Species			
	Cattle	Rats	Humans	Cats
Epinephrine	56	175	64	73
Norepinephrine	152	509	203	603
Dopamine	91	84	84	276

Source: Buhler *et al.* (1978).

stimulate metabolic and cardiovascular events. Dopamine acts primarily within the brain, via specific dopamine receptors and is not considered a hormone. Circulating concentrations of norepinephrine and dopamine are, in most mammals, considered to result from 'spillover' into the blood during sympathetic activation.

Catecholamines function as the primary mediators of the response to real or perceived stress from internal or external sources. The direct connection of the adrenal medulla to the CNS means that these compounds are rapidly released in response to external stressors. The release of catecholamines from the adrenal medulla serves to integrate the CNS and SNS with the endocrine system. The pathway involved in the stimulation of release of the catecholamines from the adrenal medulla is shown in Fig. 10.4.

In response to events that reduce blood glucose, such as sudden stress, fasting and exercise, epinephrine acts to rapidly mobilize energy reserves by increasing glycogenolysis and gluconeogenesis in the liver and glycogenolysis in skeletal muscle. This results in a rapid increase in blood glucose. Epinephrine treatment also suppresses pancreatic insulin release and induces glucagon secretion. These effects combine to assure that a high level of blood glucose is maintained for use as an energy source. In addition, lipolysis of adipose tissue is enhanced, providing free fatty acids and glycerol that can be metabolized for energy production or used to produce additional glucose by the process of gluconeogenesis.

Adrenergic Receptors

Like all hormones, catecholamines act through specific receptors on their target tissues. The receptors for catecholamines are complex, seven transmembrane domain, G-protein-linked membrane receptors which exist in several forms. The two fundamental types of adrenergic receptors are called α and β receptors. These receptors are present in many tissues and their proportions relative to one another determine the tissue response to adrenergic stimulation. α-Adrenergic receptors, in general, increase smooth muscle contraction in response to stimulation. The relative sensitivity of α receptors

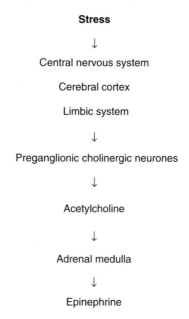

Fig. 10.4. Control of epinephrine release from the adrenal glands.

to adrenergic agents is epinephrine > norepinephrine > isoproterenol (a synthetic β-agonist). α-receptors are further subdivided into α1 and α2 subtypes. α1 receptors mediate vasoconstriction, acting through G-proteins and the phosphoinositides IP_3 and DAG, resulting in the release of calcium within the cell. α2 receptors are present in the presynaptic terminal axon of sympathetic neurones. These act as negative feedback receptors, which inhibit synaptic norepinephrine release.

While the α-receptors mediate synaptic events within the SNS, vasoconstriction and smooth muscle contraction, the predominant receptors for adrenergic agents are the β-adrenergic receptors. In general, these receptors induce smooth muscle relaxation and β-adrenergic receptors are more sensitive to epinephrine than norepinephrine. The β-adrenergic receptor isoforms are 64 kDa receptors, which are indistinguishable by immunological methods, share about 50% amino acid homologies, but have distinct functions. Ligand binding to the β receptor activates the enzyme adenylate cyclase, which catalyses the conversion of ATP to cAMP in the cytoplasm (Fig. 10.5). cAMP binds to PKA, activating this enzyme. PKA, in turn, phosphorylates and activates several cytoplasmic proteins, including hormone-sensitive lipase, the rate-limiting enzyme that catalyses triacylglycerol degradation in the adipocyte. In addition, activated PKA phosphorylates the cAMP response element binding protein (CREBP). CREBP binds to the cAMP

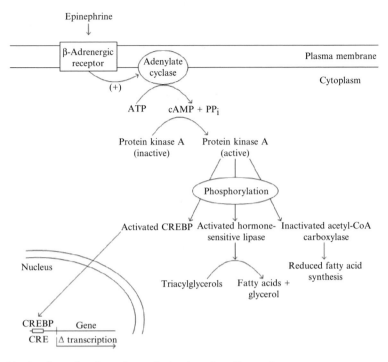

Fig. 10.5. Mechanism of action of catecholamines in adipose tissue.

response element in the regulatory portion of affected genes, where it activates gene transcription. PKA phosphorylation of other proteins results in their inactivation. For example, ACC, the rate-limiting enzyme for fatty acid synthesis, is inactivated by phosphorylation. Overall, these effects enhance lipolysis while reducing lipogenesis.

The β-adrenergic receptors are subdivided into three subtypes: β1, β2 and β3 receptors. β1 receptors mediate lipolysis in adipose tissue and other effects in the cardiac muscle and intestinal smooth muscle. They respond equally to circulating epinephrine and neural norepinephrine but are considered to be the primary neural system adrenergic receptor. They are the most abundant subtype of β-adrenergic receptor in most tissues, and account for about 80% of adipose tissue β receptors, 70% of heart, 65% of lung, 60% of skeletal muscle and 50% of liver.

β2 receptors are the major receptors for circulating epinephrine and mediate bronchodilation, vasodilation, uterine smooth muscle relaxation and glycogenolysis in the liver. They are also thought to be essential in mediating the response to β-agonists in skeletal muscle. In contrast to the β1 receptors, epinephrine is much more effective in stimulating β2 receptors than norepinephrine, which interacts weakly with the β2 receptor.

β-3 adrenergic receptors are the least abundant of the receptor subtypes. In humans and pigs, the β3 receptors constitute less than 10% of the β-adrenergic receptor subtypes in adipose tissue and are less than 2% of the β-adrenergic receptors in other tissues. In rodents, however, the β3 receptor is the predominant subtype present in white and brown adipose tissue. The β3 receptor is believed to mediate thermogenesis and lipolysis in rodent adipose tissues. This complex system of five receptors results in a very fine-tuned system in which tissues with multiple adrenergic receptors respond in accordance with the ratio of α to β receptors present in the specific tissue.

β-Adrenergic agonists

Several β-adrenergic agents have been synthesized which interact with β receptors. Some synthetic chemicals bind to β-adrenergic receptors and do not elicit a response, but block the effects of the receptor. These are termed β-receptor antagonists. Other synthetic chemicals bind to specific β-adrenergic receptors and mimic the effects of catecholamines. These are the β-receptor agonists, or β-agonists for short. In human and veterinary medicine, β-agonists are used as bronchodilators to treat asthma, to stimulate cardiac contraction strength or rate and to induce uterine relaxation. β-Agonists are active when given orally and can be used as feed supplements in animal production systems. The compounds used in farm animal production have enhanced effects on skeletal muscle and white adipose tissue and, at the doses used, have reduced effects on the cardiovascular system. β-Agonists used in animal production systems are called 'repartitioning agents' due to their effects on redirecting nutrients for use by skeletal muscle at the expense of adipose tissue. β-Agonists are effective, to varying degrees, in several species including chickens, swine, sheep and cattle. In general, they are more effective in cattle and sheep than in swine and induce better responses in swine than in poultry.

Examples of synthetic β-agonists are shown in Fig. 10.6. These include isoproterenol, a potent β-agonist that interacts with both β1 and β2 receptors better than the naturally occurring catecholamines. Clenbuterol and cimaterol are β2-agonists. Clenbuterol is used to induce bronchodilation in horses and reduce uterine contraction in pregnant cows, but is not used as a repartitioning agent in food animals. Ractopamine is a synthetic β-adrenergic receptor agonist that interacts with both β1- and β2-adrenergic receptors. Ractopamine was the first β-agonist to be approved for use in meat animals as a production enhancer, when it was approved by the FDA for use in swine in 2000, under Elanco's trade name of Paylean®. In 2003 it was approved for use in finishing cattle, under the trade name of Optaflexx®.

Effects of β-adrenergic agonists on growth and body composition

When used as feed supplements in farm animals, β-agonists increase rate of weight gain, improve feed efficiency, reduce fatness and increase carcass protein deposition of treated animals (Fig. 10.7). The effects of β-agonists on

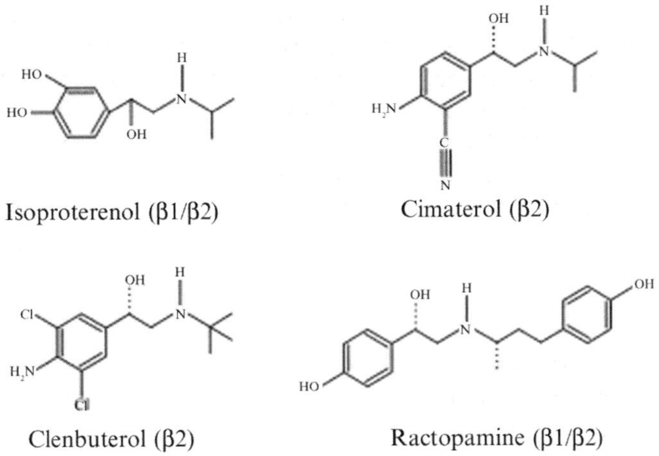

Fig. 10.6. Examples of β-agonists and their β-adrenergic receptor specificity.

animal production are species-specific and depend upon the β-agonist used. These effects are thought to be due to direct actions upon the tissues of interest, skeletal muscle and adipose tissue. Treatment with β-agonists has no effect on circulating hormones and β-adrenergic receptors in tissues affected by β-agonists are believed to mediate the effects of β-agonists.

	Species			
Parameter	Sheep	Cattle	Pigs	Chicken
Feed intake	+2	−5	−5	−
Feed efficiency	+15	+15	+5	+2
Weight gain	+15	+10	+4	+2
Muscle	+25	+10	+4	+2
Fat	−25	−30	−8	−7

Fig. 10.7. Summary of the effects of β-agonists on production characteristics in various farm animals, as percentage changes from untreated animals. Adapted from Moloney *et al.* (1991).

β-Agonists are the most potent known inducers of skeletal muscle hypertrophy. For example, treatment of lambs with clenbuterol for 2 months increases overall muscle mass by 25% to 30%, with an increase of 40% seen in the gastrocnemius muscle. This is primarily an effect on muscle hypertrophy, as there is no increase in the DNA content in affected skeletal muscles. The muscle protein accretion in response to β-agonists is due primarily to a reduction in protein degradation. A decrease in both lysosomal protease activity (cathepsin B) and in non-lysosomal proteinase activity (e.g. calpain μ) is observed with β-agonist treatment. Reduced calpain μ activity is due to an increase in the calpain inhibitor, calpastatin. Muscle hypertrophy and protein accretion is rapid and is measurable within 2 days of treatment in rats, and is specific for skeletal muscle. Cardiac and smooth muscle are unaffected. The effects on skeletal muscle are time-dependent, characterized by rapid early growth, which is later attenuated. Attenuation may be due to downregulation of β receptors in skeletal muscle. Studies in rodents show that receptor concentration is reduced by 50% after 18 days of treatment with clenbuterol. This attenuation can be avoided by intermittent treatment, e.g. treating for 2 days and resting for 2 days.

About 40% of the hogs in the USA are fed the β-agonist ractopamine (Paylean®). As with any production enhancer, animals must be provided with adequate nutrition, especially amino acids balanced in relation to lysine, to provide the increased demand for lean deposition. β-Agonists are provided as feed supplements and are most effective when given to older, heavier animals. Low doses, in parts per million, are most effective and weight gain is reduced when higher doses – more than 20 mg/kg – are fed. This is due to a reduction of appetite and lower feed intake at higher doses. Problems with metabolic acidosis and slow, downer pigs can occur. Pigs treated with ractopamine have been likened to weightlifters. They walk slowly and stiffly and take longer to load into transportation vehicles. As they are highly susceptible to stress, they must be treated gently, not crowded and not herded with electric prods.

A significant drawback to the use of β-agonists in many farm animals is the increased toughness, as measured by Warner–Bratzler shear force, of the resulting meat products. This is especially prominent in treated lambs, in which the toughness of meat is more than doubled compared to non-treated animals. Chickens and cattle are less affected, but still show a 15% to 35% decrease in muscle tenderness. The tenderness of meat of ractopamine-treated pigs is unaffected by treatment. The effects of β-agonists are specific for muscle fibre type, consistently increasing the cross-sectional area of Type II (fast, white, glycolytic) fibres, while the trophic effects of β-agonists on Type I fibres (slow, red, oxidative) are inconsistent. When animals are treated for long periods with β-agonists, there is a switch of fibre types, from Type I to Type II. The long-term implications of this alteration of fibre type are unknown. The effects of β-agonists on skeletal muscle are thought to be mediated by the β2 receptor, the predominant adrenergic receptor in skeletal muscle.

References and Further Reading

Buhler, H.U., Da Prada, M., Haefely, W. and Picotti, G.B. (1978) Plasma adrenaline, noradrenaline and dopamine in man and different animal species. *Journal of Physiology (London)* 276, 311–326.

Etherton, T.D. and Smith, S.B. (1991) Somatotropin and β-adrenergic agonists: their efficacy and mechanisms of action. *Journal of Animal Science* 69 (Suppl. 2), 2–26.

Hadley, M.E. (2000) Catecholamines and the sympathoadrenal system. In: *Endocrinology*, 5th edn. Prentice-Hall, Upper Saddle River, New Jersey, pp. 338–361.

Mersmann, H.J. (1998) Overview of the effects of β-adrenergic receptor agonists on animal growth including mechanisms of action. *Journal of Animal Science* 76, 160–172.

Moloney, A., Allen, P., Joseph, R. and Tarrant, V. (1991) Influence of beta-adrenergic agonists and similar compounds on growth. In: Pearson, A.M. and Dutson, T.R. (eds) *Growth Regulation in Farm Animals*, Vol. 7. Elsevier Applied Science, New York, pp. 455–513.

Moody, D.E., Hancock, D.L. and Hancock, D.B. (2000) Phenethanolamine repartitioning agents. In: D'Mello, J.P.F. (ed.) *Farm Animal Metabolism and Nutrition*. CAB International, Wallingford, UK, pp. 65–96.

Stock, M.J. and Rothwell, N.J. (1986) Effects of β-adrenergic agonists on metabolism and body composition. In: Buttery, P.J., Haynes, N.B. and Lindsay, D.B. (eds) *Control and Manipulation of Animal Growth*. Butterworths, London, pp. 249–257.

Stoller, G.M., Zerby, H.N., Moeller, S.J., Baas, T.J., Johnson, C. and Watkins, L.E. (2003) The effect of feeding ractopamine (Paylean) on muscle quality and sensory characteristics in three diverse genetic lines of swine. *Journal of Animal Science* 81, 1508–1516.

11 Leptin, Body Composition and Appetite Control

Regulation of food intake, metabolism and body composition is of prime importance to farm animal producers. Animals do not thrive without adequate feed intake, and those that do not efficiently utilize feed intake are not economically competitive. Animals that are overly fat or lean are unprofitable for producers and unacceptable to consumers. Much of an animal producer's effort and resources are directed towards providing adequate nutrition to his animals and small alterations in feed consumption and efficiency are important in providing an economical return on invested resources. Thus, the control of feed intake, the subsequent utilization of nutrients and the ultimate production of a desirable meat product are linked. The regulation of appetite at the cellular, molecular and endocrine levels is only now being understood and utilized by animal producers.

In a broad perspective, food preferences are largely innate (genetic) in animals. Carnivores, of course, are not physiologically adapted to digest, absorb and flourish on a high roughage vegetarian diet, while herbivores have not evolved to survive on a high protein, meat-based diet. Nevertheless, within bounds, food preferences are also a learned behaviour. Animals can be taught the avoidance of certain foods, either as a result of sickness from consuming a toxic substance or in the laboratory by behavioural modification. Likewise, food that produces pleasurable sensations to the animal is readily consumed. Learned food consumption is especially evident in omnivores such as humans, who have a wide range of diet options, from vegan to vegetarian to carnivorous. In developed countries, frequently these preferences are a result of parental guidance or pressure from peers or commercial sources and are thus learned, not innate. Geographical circumstances also play a large role in the selection and consumption of foods. As an extreme, the diet of an Inuit, for example, consists primarily of protein and fat, derived from fish and marine mammals, with essentially no vegetables. More temperate latitudes provide a more diversified diet.

Ingestion of food is a complex process, regulated by sensory, mechanical, chemical, hormonal and neural mechanisms. The consumption of food is a result of an initial positive sensory evaluation (Fig. 11.1). This includes the sight and smell of the food, followed by oral evaluation through mastication. This provides additional sensory inputs, including the food's texture

©K.L. Hossner 2005. *Hormonal Regulation of Farm Animal Growth* (K.L. Hossner)

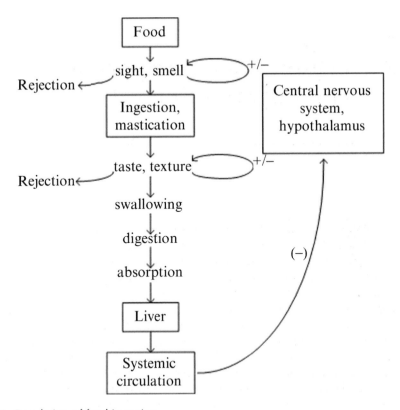

Fig. 11.1. Regulation of food ingestion.

and taste. The food can be rejected at this point. If it is not, the food is swallowed, digested and absorbed into the body by the gastrointestinal tract. Lipids are absorbed into the lymphatic system, while protein and carbohydrate (or VFA in ruminants) nutrients are taken directly into the bloodstream. Most of these blood-borne nutrients are absorbed into the hepatic portal system where they are transported to the liver for oxidation and energy production or transformed into storage products.

The induction of feeding behaviour and feed intake and the cessation of this process when the animal is full (satiety) maintains the animal's energy balance and ensures metabolic homeostasis. Energy intake, in the form of nutrients, is correlated with body weight. Reduced food intake results in an increase in energy expenditure as animals increase the oxidation of substrates via intermediary metabolism in an effort to maintain body weight. Excess food energy is efficiently converted into fat stores. At the same time, oxidation of energy reserves is reduced. These responses to excess energy availability result from evolutionary adaptations that favour energy storage over dissipation. This provides a survival advantage for animals in the wild. These animals, unlike domesticated animals, undergo sporadic periods of fasting when food is scarce or unavailable. During times of food scarcity, animals derive their energy from the metabolism of fat stores that were accumulated during periods of food abundance. Survival mechanisms that favour energy storage, weight gain and fat accumulation predominate, while there are few mechanisms that favour the loss of body weight. Thus, the development of fatness in animals and obesity in humans is due to the evolutionary advantages of excess food consumption and storage.

It should be emphasized at the outset that the regulation of appetite, food-seeking or food-aversive behaviour and food intake are all processes that are ultimately regulated by the CNS, and specifically, the hypothalamus. It has long been known that specific areas of the hypothalamus, the ARC nucleus, the ventromedial hypothalamus (VMH) and the lateral hypothalamus (LH), regulate feeding and satiety. Destruction of the VMH leads to hyperphagia and obesity, while lesions in the ARC or LH induce anorexia and weight loss. These observations suggested that there were specific, distinct feeding and satiety centres in the hypothalamus, but more refined studies support a more diffuse integration of food intake and satiety. Inputs into the CNS may be neural, nutrient-mediated or hormonal and the regulation of appetite and thus energy homeostasis can be acute or chronic. The focus of this chapter is on the hormonal control of long-term energy homeostasis by the adipose hormone leptin, but we will first discuss the factors that have traditionally been studied as short-term regulators of food intake.

Theories on the Short-term Regulation of Food Intake

Over the past half-century, many theories of the control of food intake have been proposed. One of the earliest was *the thermostatic theory* of Brobeck (1948), which proposed that animals eat to maintain a constant body temperature. This was shown to be true only in special circumstances, e.g. to avoid hypothermia. In 1953, Mayer proposed *the glucostat theory*, which suggested that the concentrations of glucose in the bloodstream played a negative feedback role in feed intake. This was supported by the correlation of satiety and elevated blood glucose concentrations after a meal. In addition, glucose infusion into monogastric animals reduced feed intake, although glucose infusion had no effect on ruminant feed intake. It is now known that specific regions of the hypothalamus that control feeding are sensitive to changes in glucose concentrations and glucose, either directly, or indirectly, through insulin or leptin, plays a significant role in the acute regulation of feed intake in monogastrics. In ruminants, the products of microbial carbohydrate metabolism, the VFAs, subsume the role of glucose.

Mechanical and chemical properties of food also play a role in the regulation of food intake. This is especially important in ruminants, which due to the large reservoir of feed in the rumen are subject to the inhibitory effects of gut-fill. In this case, the physical capacity of the rumen determines, to some extent, the feeding behaviour and food intake of the animal. Animals with a full rumen have reduced feed intake. As the rumen empties, feed intake increases. This effect is not strictly physical, but also depends upon the chemical and osmotic properties of the consumed food and thus likely involves chemical sensing via chemoreceptors as well as the mechanoreceptors of the gut. The physical effects of gut fill are mediated by stretch receptors in the rumen, but the effects of feed composition suggest that nutritional and hormonal mechanisms are also involved. This is, like the regulation by blood glucose and insulin, a short-term regulatory mechanism.

The Long-term Regulation of Food Intake – the Lipostat Theory

The early theories discussed above on the short-term regulation of eating were shaped by the scientific environment of the times. Thus, what may seem to us as the somewhat obvious effects of 'being full', or body temperature and circulating glucose concentrations were based on factors that were known at the time to be involved in regulating food intake. While all of these theories are still valid to some extent, they apply primarily to the acute regulation of food ingestion. *The lipostat theory* was proposed by Kennedy in 1953 to explain the regulation of long-term energy homeostasis and food intake. This theory postulated that the body's energy stores, in the form of fat, were somehow affected by the CNS, which regulated energy homeostasis, the balance between energy consumption, use and storage. The observation that stores of body fat are almost constant in young animals indicated that long-term food intake is precisely regulated. Kennedy suggested that, as opposed to a direct neural pathway that might regulate fat deposition, circulating metabolites were the most likely candidates to regulate long-term food intake. In contrast to the short-term regulation of food intake by factors such as blood glucose, insulin and gut fill, the lipostat was postulated as a system that modulates a slower response to deficits in whole-animal energy reserves. Thus, when energy reserves, in the form of adipose tissue, were high, the satiety centres in the hypothalamus were activated and food intake was reduced. During fasting and starvation, adipose reserves are mobilized for energy, and appetite increases concurrently.

Evidence for the lipostat theory was provided by several studies using the technique of parabiosis. In this method, the circulatory system of two animals is surgically connected. This allows one to observe the blood-borne effects of experimental manipulation of one animal on its conjoined partner. Hervey (1959) studied the systemic effects of an obese rat on a conjoined normal rat (Fig. 11.2). To induce obesity, he destroyed the VMH region. This area of the hypothalamus inhibits food intake. Its destruction induced hyperphagia (excessive eating) and, subsequently, obesity. He then surgically joined these obese, hyperphagic rats in parabiosis with normal rats. The normal rats stopped eating and lost weight. This provided strong evidence that some factor in the circulation (a 'satiety signal') from the obese rat was affecting the VMH of the normal rat to reduce food intake. Later studies by other scientists in the 1980s showed that this satiety factor mediated feeding in other models of obesity. Thus, rats with diet-induced obesity parabiosed with non-obese rats reduced the food intake of the normal rats.

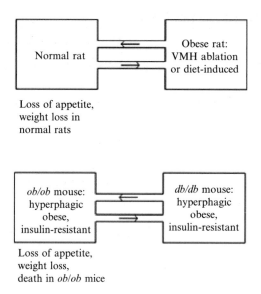

Loss of appetite,
weight loss in
normal rats

Loss of appetite,
weight loss,
death in *ob/ob* mice

Fig. 11.2. Effects of parabiosis on feed intake and body weight in rodents.

The body weight loss of the normal rats was due to a selective reduction in body fat. This was attributed to an 'energy stabilizing' factor that regulated energy homeostasis in the body that was carried in the circulation from the obese to the normal rat. These elegant whole-animal experiments led to the conclusion that regulation of appetite (and thus body energy reserves in the form of fat) was likely mediated by a blood-borne factor, either a hormone or a metabolite, which acted at the level of the hypothalamus.

To examine this phenomenon further, two widely used animal models for diabetes and obesity, the diabetic mouse (*db/db*) and the obese mouse (*ob/ob*), were used. It was known that these strains were the result of single gene mutations, although the identity of the affected genes was unknown. Thus, these animals provided excellent models with which to examine single gene effects on humoral-mediated food intake and obesity. Both strains of mice exhibit the characteristics of Type II (insulin-resistant) diabetes and are obese, hyperphagic, hyperglycaemic and hyperinsulinaemic. When the *db/db* and *ob/ob* mice were joined in parabiosis, the *ob/ob* mice became anorexic, hypoglycaemic and died of starvation. This suggested that the two strains of mice had defects in different genes, which resulted in a similar phenotype. In addition, the results suggested that the *db/db* mice produced a blood-borne factor that was absent in the *ob/ob* mice which inhibits food intake. Thus, the *ob/ob* mice react to a 'satiety signal', which is produced by the *db/db* mice but is ineffective in the *db/db* mice. It is now known that the *ob/ob* mice are leptin-deficient and the *db/db* mice produce leptin but have no functional leptin receptors. These observations set the stage for the discovery of leptin, a blood-borne satiety factor that regulates long-term energy homeostasis (Table 11.1).

Table 11.1. Factors that regulate food intake.

Short-term signals	Short-term responses
A. Sensory inputs: sight, smell, taste, texture, memory	Size, duration, frequency of meals
B. Nutrient inputs: glucose, fatty acids,	Ingestion, digestion, absorption of nutrients amino acids
C. Gut signals: chemoreceptors, mechanoreceptors, gut hormones	Food-induced thermogenesis
Long-term signals	Long-term responses
Circulating nutrients, hormones and metabolites	Hunger/satiety
	Glycogen, lipid energy storage
	Thermogenesis, energy expenditure

The Discovery of Leptin

Dr Friedman's group at Rockefeller University used the *ob/ob* mouse and sophisticated molecular biology techniques to search for and eventually isolate the product of the obese gene. In 1994, Friedman and his colleagues reported the positional cloning and characterization of the obese gene from white adipose tissue of the *ob/ob* mice. Friedman showed that in the *ob/ob* mice this gene contained a mutation that interrupts the transcription of the *ob* gene product, resulting in a biologically inactive molecule. The absence of the product of this gene in *ob/ob* mice was responsible for overeating and obesity in these mice. The natural product of this gene in wild-type mice was dubbed leptin (from the Greek word *leptos*, meaning thin). Leptin treatment of the *ob/ob* mice reduced feed intake and lowered body weights. The reduction in body weight occurred specifically through a selective loss of fat mass. The circulating levels of this hormone were highly correlated with fat mass. Thus, leptin fulfilled the role of the long-sought 'lipostat', proposed by Kennedy, a humoral factor that was proportional to fat mass and regulated energy homeostasis and food intake (Fig. 11.3). Not unimportantly, this was also the first indication that adipose tissue acted not only as a passive energy storage depot, but also as an endocrine organ, secreting a satiety factor that regulated food intake and energy homeostasis. Leptin is believed to be an important regulator of appetite, energy metabolism and body composition, essential factors in efficient farm animal production.

The leptin gene and molecule

The *ob* gene, which codes for leptin, consists of 4500 bp. A nonsense mutation at position 105 of the gene interrupts the transcription of the *ob* gene in

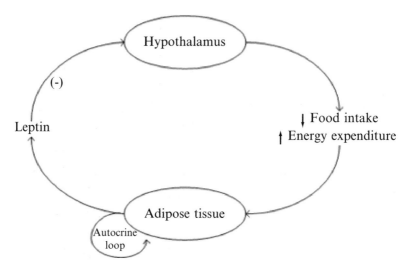

Fig. 11.3. The production and effects of leptin.

ob/ob mice and produces a truncated, biologically inactive molecule in these animals. The leptin molecule is a single-chain polypeptide containing 146 amino acids and circulates as a 16,000 Da peptide. The molecule is highly conserved and displays an 84% amino acid sequence identity between mice and humans. Leptin is synthesized and secreted primarily by white adipose tissue. The leptin gene has been cloned from several domestic animal species, including pigs, cattle, sheep and chickens.

Leptin receptors and binding proteins

The receptors for leptin are members of the Class I cytokine receptor family. They consist of a single protein chain that traverses the plasma membrane (Fig. 11.4). Ligand binding induces dimerization and activation of the receptor. Five isoforms of the leptin receptor exist, composed of 830 to 1162 amino acids, and are designated Ob-Ra through Ob-Re. The isoforms are derived from different splicing of a single gene and differ from one another in their overall length and the extent of their cytoplasmic domain. Only one of these receptors, Ob-Rb, contains all domains, extracellular, transmembrane and intracellular, needed for a fully active receptor. The Ob-Rb receptor is believed to mediate leptin's effects on appetite and food intake. This receptor contains the Box 1 and Box 2 motifs that are important for signal transduction via the JAK/STAT pathway. Box 1 serves as a binding site for JAK2, while Box 2 binds STAT3. The Ob-Rb receptor is found in low levels in many tissues of the body, but is especially abundant in specific nuclei of the hypothalamus that are involved in feeding and satiety. The ARC nucleus, the VMH and the paraventricular nucleus (PVN) all contain the Ob-Rb receptor,

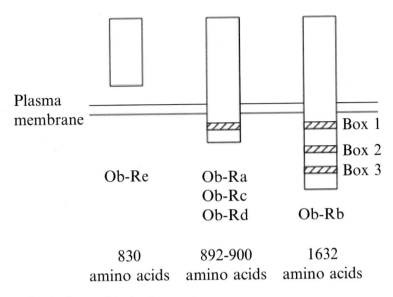

Fig. 11.4. Molecular forms of the leptin receptors.

marking these feeding and satiety centres as the hypothalamic targets of leptin. Many of the CNS-mediated effects of leptin are mediated by interaction with the ARC nucleus. The ARC nucleus is the site of synthesis of the neurotransmitter, neuropeptide Y (NPY). NPY is potent inducer of appetite and food intake. The primary effect of leptin on the inhibition of feeding is believed to be via the inhibition of the synthesis and release of NPY by the ARC. The Ob-Rb receptor is also found in the LH, a region considered to be involved in feeding, not satiety. Finally, the Ob-Rb receptor is found in the dorsomedial nucleus (DMN) of the hypothalamus. This region contains neurones that have complex autonomic effects on long-term growth and body composition. More recent evidence suggests that the appetite-suppressing effects of leptin may involve hypothalamic αMSH, agouti-related protein (AGRP) and melanin-concentrating hormone (MCH). These hypothalamic neurotransmitters are discussed at the end of this chapter.

The truncated receptor forms, Ob-Ra, Ob-Rc and Ob-Rd, have a shortened intracellular domain, consisting of 32 to 40 amino acids. These isoforms are found in many tissues, including skeletal muscle, adipose, kidney, liver and the choroid plexus but a role for these short isoforms in regulating appetite has not been demonstrated. The Ob-Ra receptor is abundant in the choroid plexus of the brain and may act as a transport protein for leptin, allowing entry into the CNS, bypassing the blood–brain barrier. This truncated receptor also exists in the kidney, where it is thought to play a role in the clearance of leptin. Leptin has many direct effects on peripheral tissues. Whether these effects are mediated by the truncated receptors or by the small amounts of Ob-Rb present in the tissues is unclear. The last short receptor form, Ob-Re, is a soluble receptor, lacking the transmembrane and cytoplasmic domains. It consists of only a 830-amino acid, extracellular, ligand-binding domain. This receptor is found in the circulation, where it acts as a binding protein for leptin. In addition, Ob-Re is found in the placenta and increases to 40-fold during pregnancy, leading the hypothesis that it is involved in regulating fetal growth and energy use.

Mutations in the leptin receptor that result in a reduction of leptin receptors or in non-functional receptors have been shown to be responsible for obesity in laboratory animals. Just as the absence of leptin itself results in overeating, obesity and diabetes, animals with defects in leptin receptors display a similar phenotype. Although circulating leptin concentrations are elevated, these animals are unable to respond to leptin and are leptin-resistant. For example, the genetic diabetic mice (*db/db*), discussed above, have only the truncated Ob-Ra form of the leptin receptor. The obese strain of rats, Zucker fatty rats (*fa/fa*), have low numbers of leptin receptors due to a single amino acid substitution in the receptor molecule.

Like the IGFs, circulating leptin is complexed to serum-binding proteins in a specific, saturable and reversible manner. Rodents have three circulating binding proteins with molecular masses of 85, 176 and 240 kDa, while humans have two binding proteins with masses of 176 and 240 kDa. It appears that leptin binding to these proteins is regulated by physiological processes. Obesity reduces the proportion of bound leptin, providing more unbound, presumably active leptin, while fasting increases protein-bound leptin binding.

Biological actions of leptin

The biological effects of the leptin have been examined in the obese diabetic mouse models, *ob/ob*, *db/db* and wild-type mice. When injected into the leptin-deficient *ob/ob* mice, leptin rapidly (4 days) reduced food intake to about 40% of the untreated *ob/ob* mice and reduced their body weight by about 40% after 33 days of treatment. Pair-fed *ob/ob* mice, matched by age, sex and weight, lost less weight than animals treated with leptin. Leptin treatment of *db/db* mice did not affect food intake or body weight and later studies of *db/db* mice showed them to lack the leptin receptor. Treatment of wild-type mice with leptin resulted in a small, but significant loss in body weight of approximately 12% and food intake of about 10%. As might be expected, these effects required higher doses of leptin than those that were effective in the leptin-deficient *ob/ob* mice. Body weight loss in the leptin-treated *ob/ob* mice was due to an almost exclusive loss of adipose tissue mass. The lean body masses of control and leptin-treated mice were not different from one another. In wild-type mice body fat was reduced from 12.2% to 0.67% by leptin treatment. These early studies demonstrated the effectiveness of leptin in reducing food intake, body weight and, specifically, the fat mass of leptin-deficient and normal mice. The effects of leptin on appetite that are mediated via the hypothalamus are indirect, and act through a reduction of hypothalamic neurotransmitter NPY. Leptin effects that are mediated by NPY include a reduction of food intake, body weight and fat mass in normal and leptin-deficient animals, induction of puberty in mice and increased thermogenesis.

In light of the effects of leptin on body fat and appetite, the effects of leptin on energy metabolism were examined. When injected into *ob/ob* mice, leptin induced increased oxygen consumption, locomotor activity and body temperature of these obese mice to values seen in wild-type mice. In addition, the elevated serum insulin and glucose values in these animals were decreased to near-normal values in a dose-dependent manner by leptin treatment. None of these parameters was affected by leptin treatment of wild-type mice. Thus, leptin administration reversed the physiological problems associated with the obese phenotype, including endocrine and energy homeostasis parameters.

In addition, injection of small amounts of leptin (60 pmol) directly into the third ventricle of the brain, where it has direct access to the hypothalamus, induced a rapid (within 30 min) reduction of food intake and increased oxygen consumption in lean and *ob/ob* mice. These very rapid-onset effects of leptin on oxygen consumption indicated that the sympathetic nervous system (SNS) may be involved, and the effects of norepinephrine on brown adipose tissue metabolism may mediate these effects of leptin.

The effects of leptin on thermogenesis and oxygen consumption may be mediated via the hypothalamus and sympathetic innervation or may be a result of direct effects of leptin on peripheral tissues. The thermogenic effects of leptin are likely mediated by mitochondrial UCPs. The UCPs uncouple oxidative phosphorylation from ATP generation and increase proton leakage through the inner mitochondrial membrane. Instead of using the proton energy of the cytochrome chain for oxidative phosphorylation, the energy is released as heat, resulting in increased thermogenesis. Different UCPs have been found in various tissues. Brown adipose tissue contains UCP-1, while homologous proteins called UCP-2 and UCP-3 have been reported. Several mammalian tissues containing UCP-2 and UCP-3 are expressed primarily in skeletal muscle. Leptin directly induces expression of UCP-2 in pancreatic islets and in epididymal, retroperitoneal and subcutaneous fat of normal rats. Leptin administered intracerebroventricularly (ICV) also stimulated UCP mRNA by 70% in rat brown adipose tissue. Leptin treatment of *ob/ob* mice stimulated UCP-3 expression in skeletal muscle. Thus, leptin has important effects on energy metabolism in animals, increasing oxygen consumption and motor activity, increasing thermogenesis by direct induction of mitochondrial UCPs and by indirect actions through the CNS and the SNS.

In all studies to date, leptin is more effective in the leptin-deficient *ob/ob* animals than in normal animals. In addition, even the highest doses of leptin used did not induce a 'supranormal' response. That is, the animals' metabolic indices, insulin and glucose levels did not exceed normal levels and the values of wild-type mice were largely unaffected. Most obesity in humans is diet-induced, and as a result, obese humans have elevated leptin, proportional to their fat mass. As a result, most obese humans have plenty of leptin and are actually leptin-resistant.

Effects of leptin on reproduction

A long held tenet of reproductive biology is that adequate energy stores, in the form of adipose tissue, are required for efficient reproduction. Adequate energy reserves are needed to support the growth and development of the embryo and fetus, parturition and lactation. It is axiomatic in farm animal production systems that lean females (poor body condition) reproduce less efficiently than those with moderate body fat. In human athletes, lean women have a delayed onset of puberty and the reproductive cycles of lean females are interrupted. As leptin levels are proportional to body fat, it was hypothesized that leptin may act as the signal to the reproductive system that sufficient body fat exists to support a successful conception and pregnancy. Leptin treatment of normal female mice induces early puberty, reproductive system maturation and mating. Leptin does this by inducing release of the reproductive hormones LH and FSH, acting directly on the anterior pituitary and indirectly, inducing LHRH release by the hypothalamus. Leptin has similar effects in the food-restricted, infertile *ob/ob* male mouse, inducing testicular maturation and normal fertility. Embryonic and fetal leptin concentrations increase during development and are proportional to fetal size and birth weight. Leptin and leptin receptor mRNA is present in human placental tissue. These observations suggest that leptin may be involved in placental–uterine–fetal growth and development and may act locally or in a hormonal fashion to signal nutrient availability and metabolic regulation of the fetoplacental unit during embryonic development.

Direct peripheral effects of leptin

In addition to those effects of leptin that are mediated by the hypothalamus, leptin has several direct effects on a variety of tissues. Direct effects of a hormone or growth factor are difficult to establish using animal models injected with the factor of choice, *in vivo*. Even if carefully controlled, whole animal studies are generally ambiguous, due to the multiple interactions of the exogenous drug with the myriad of regulatory systems in the living animal. For this reason, studies using cells *in vitro* are performed to negate extraneous factors under defined conditions. For example, leptin can act as a mitogen, stimulating the proliferation of mouse embryonic fibroblast cells, *in vitro*. Leptin has direct effects on white adipose tissue, where it acts through the Ob-Rb receptor. Leptin suppresses the expression of adipocyte ACC, an enzyme required for lipogenesis, while stimulating lipolysis. In C2C12 cells, leptin stimulates glucose transport and glycogen synthesis at physiological levels. Leptin also stimulates pancreatic islet UCP-2 mRNA, mRNA for enzymes involved with free fatty acid oxidation, and inhibits fatty acid esterification. In the reproductive system, leptin has direct effects on inducing the release of FSH and LH from anterior pituitaries and LHRH release from the hypothalamus *in vitro*.

Recent studies have shown that both long and short forms of the leptin receptors are present in haematopoietic organs, endothelial cells and keratinocytes. In haematopoietic cells, leptin induces cell survival, proliferation and differentiation. In endothelial cells, leptin stimulates the formation of new blood vessels (angiogenesis) and the local expression of leptin and its receptors in the ovary, uterine endometrium and placenta has led to suggestions that leptin may be involved in the extensive vascularization/devascularization that occurs in these tissues during the reproductive cycle and pregnancy. Leptin is also involved in stimulating the proliferation of keratinocytes during skin repair and is thought to be involved in wound healing. There are high levels of leptin and the leptin receptor in fetal bone and cartilage. Leptin, acting via the CNS, and probably locally, inhibits bone formation and *ob/ob* mice have high bone masses.

The direct effects of leptin on many different tissues suggest that this hormone is involved in the coordination of many physiological processes. Leptin acts not only on the hypothalamus to regulate food intake, but also acts as a peripheral hormone and as a local autocrine and paracrine growth factor in its own right.

Regulation of leptin concentrations

Circulating concentrations of leptin are modulated by several physiological states. As we have seen, the concentration of circulating leptin is proportional to fat mass. Leptin mRNA concentrations are higher in subcutaneous fat than in omental fat. Leptin concentrations are reduced by fasting and by the antidiabetic drugs, the TZDs. Leptin concentrations are sexually dimorphic, and are increased in females, independent of adiposity. When fat mass is accounted for, females have about twice the amount of circulating leptin than males. Leptin concentrations vary diurnally and are higher at night than during the daytime. The hormones insulin, glucocorticoids and GH induce an increase in leptin. As might be expected nutritional status affects leptin concentrations, and a chronic high fat diet increases circulating levels of leptin. Leptin is elevated during pregnancy. Testosterone and chronic GH lower leptin levels. The physiological conditions of exercise, cold exposure and cold-induced feed intake have no effect on leptin concentrations.

Significance of leptin to animal production

One may wonder about the significance to animal production of a hormone that reduces appetite, body weight and feed intake. The discovery of leptin provided the first link between the systemic circulation and the CNS that regulated long-term energy balance. As the CNS is a protected site, entrance into this sanctuary is highly regulated and limited to a select few. This ensures the protection of the CNS from the myriad of toxins, metabolites and environmental chemical challenges encountered on a daily basis. A naturally occurring circulating hormone that can pass through the blood–brain barrier and alter feeding behaviour is of immense importance.

Leptin's effects on animal energy metabolism are not in keeping with efficient animal production. As leptin increases oxygen consumption, and thus thermogenesis and metabolic rate, by uncoupling oxidative phosphorylation, the use of leptin or leptin agonists for animal production is counterintuitive. To make use of leptin's potential effects on energy metabolism, the use of leptin antagonists, which block the effects of leptin, would be beneficial. A leptin mutant, consisting of a single amino acid alteration, has been described. This antagonist induces weight gain in mice and may provide the advantages of quicker growth and earlier fat deposition in economically important animals. Studies to identify small molecules that are orally active, cross the blood–brain barrier and antagonize the effects of leptin are being explored for use in production animals.

The effects of leptin on reproductive system processes are striking. The communication of adipose tissue with the reproductive system via leptin is unique and complete as it involves all portions of the reproductive system: hypothalamus, pituitary, ovaries and testes. In addition, leptin may be involved in regulation of fetal, placental and uterine metabolism and angiogenesis. Leptin's broad effects on reproduction and embryonic development endow it with a true reproductive hormone status. Leptin may be useful to induce early puberty in slightly thinner, younger animals and may be used to shorten the interval from parturition to oestrus. These effects, as well as possible role in fetal growth and development, may enhance the reproductive efficiency of farm animals.

Appetite-inducing (Orexigenic) Peptides of the Hypothalamus

Appetite is highly regulated in vertebrates and chemically coded in the hypothalamus. The hypothalamus consists of a neural network of appetite-inducing (orexigenic) and appetite-inhibiting (anorexigenic) signals which are modulated by nutrients, neural stimuli and hormones. Some of the more important hypothalamic regulators of appetite are outlined.

NPY is a major regulator of appetite and plays a role in many appetite-regulating mechanisms. NPY is thought to be the naturally occurring appetite transducer and the essential component of the final pathway in the hypothalamic integration of energy homeostasis. It is the only messenger molecule that can be considered as a physiological appetite transducer in the brain. NPY is present in the ARC and dorsomedial nuclei. Its amino acid sequence is related to pancreatic polypeptide. NPY is potent appetite stimulant, which is released in the dark in nocturnal feeding rodents and in anticipation of scheduled feeding. There is increased release during fasting. In the obese, leptin-resistant rodent models, *ob/ob* mice, *fa/fa* rats and *db/db* mice, an increase in hypothalamic NPY expression accompanies the obese, hyperphagic phenotype of these animals. NPY expression in these animals is reduced by leptin treatment. In physiological states that require increased energy resources, such as lactation, hypothalamic expression of NPY is increased, leading to increased appetite and food consumption. This provides the animal with the energy necessary to support the increased energy demand for milk synthesis.

Galanin (gal) is another peptide (29 amino acids) found throughout the hypothalamus. As NPY neurones may induce gal synthesis, gal, through β-endorphins, may mediate the effects of NPY, acting to induce epinephrine release. As there is no correlation of gal expression with daily feeding patterns and as fasting reduces gal expression, its role in the regulation of daily feeding is uncertain.

Orexins, also called hypocretins, are produced in many places in the body, including the LH, the gut, pancreas, kidney and the adrenal and thyroid glands. The orexins are the product of a single gene which produces two peptides by alternative splicing, orexin A (33 amino acids) and orexin B (28 amino acids). ICV injection of orexins increases food intake and wakefulness. ORX-A increases heart rate, blood pressure, intestinal motility and gastric acid secretion, while both orexins induce epinephrine/norepinephrine and insulin release. This suggests that orexins may play a role in the mediation of the stress response. The acute, short-term effects of orexins on feeding may be secondary to effects on wakefulness and activity. The orexigenic effects of the orexins are mediated by an induction of NPY expression. Orexins are induced by reduced blood glucose levels, while increased circulating levels of glucose and leptin reduce orexin expression. There are two receptors for the orexins. Orexin receptor mutations induce narcolepsy in dogs and humans.

Other hypothalamic peptides which are orexigenic include opioid peptides (e.g. β-endorphin), which have a short-lived modest effect, and MCH which may potentiate nocturnal feeding. Anorexic signals in the hypothalamus, which balance and antagonize orexic signals, include CRH, considered a tonic restraint of appetite, and urocortin (a CRH-related peptide), which is more potent than CRH. In addition, neurotensin, glucagon-like peptide-1, melanocortin and AGRP are potential anorexic peptides.

References and Further Reading

Auwerx, J. and Staels, B. (1998) Leptin. *The Lancet* 351, 737–742.

Conway, G.S. and Jacobs, H.S. (1997) Leptin: a hormone of reproduction. *Human Reproduction* 12, 633–635.

Flier, J.S. (1997) Leptin expression and action: new experimental paradigms. *Proceedings of the National Academy of Sciences USA* 94, 4242–4245.

Flier, J.S. and Lowell, B.B. (1997) Obesity research springs a protein leak. *Nature Genetics* 15, 223–224.

Flier, J.S. and Maratos-Flier, E. (1998) Obesity and the hypothalamus: novel peptides for new pathways. *Cell* 92, 427–440.

Frisch, R.E. and Revelle, R. (1970) Height and weight at menarche and a hypothesis of critical body weights and adolescent events. *Science* 169, 397–399.

Forbes, J.M. (1995) *Voluntary Food Intake and Diet Selection in Farm Animals.* CAB International, Wallingford, UK, 532 pp.

Friedman, J.M. (2002) The function of leptin in nutrition, weight and physiology. *Nutrition Reviews* 60, S1–S14.

Fruhbeck, G. (2002) Peripheral actions of leptin and its involvement in disease. *Nutrition Reviews* 60, S47–S55.

Harrold, J.A. (2004) Leptin leads hypothalamic feeding circuits in a new direction. *Bioessays* 26, 1043–1045.

Hervey, G.R. (1959) The effects of lesions in the hypothalamus in parabiotic rats. *Journal of Physiology (London)* 145, 336–352.

Hossner, K.L. (1998) Cellular, molecular and physiological aspects of leptin: potential application in animal production. *Canadian Journal of Animal Science* 78, 463–472.

Kennedy, G.C. (1953) The role of depot fat in the hypothalamic control of food intake in the rat. *Proceedings of the Royal Society of London* B140, 578–592.

Tartaglia, L.A. (1997) The leptin receptor. *Journal of Biological Chemistry* 272, 6093–6096.

Wilding, J.P.H. (2002) Neuropeptides and appetite control. *Diabetic Medicine* 19, 619–627.

Zhang, Y., Proenca, R., Maffei, M., Barone, M., Leopold, L. and Friedman, J.M. (1994) Positional cloning of the mouse obese gene and its human homologue. *Nature* 372, 425–431.

Index

3T3-F442A cells 164, 174, 175
3T3-L1 cells 164–165, 166, 168, 170, 171, 173, 174, 175, 176, 177
5α-reductase 183

αGPDH 78
ACC 197, 212
acetycholine 76, 193
acetyl-CoA 88, 89, 92, 167
acetyl-coenzyme A carboxylase (ACC) 84, 88, 104, 168, 174
acid phosphatase 65, 131, 133, 134
acromegaly 104
ACTH 176
actin 68, 71, 73, 74, 76, 77, 79
activin 140, 141
acyl-CoA 91
ADD1/SREBP1 167, 169, 170–172, 174
adenylate cyclase 50, 130, 196
adipoblast 84, 86
adipocyte 163, 164
adipogenesis 84, 167, 168, 169, 170, 171, 173, 176
adiponectin 178
adipose tissue 82
adipsin 166, 176
adrenal cortex 41
adrenal gland 41, 181, 191
adrenal medulla 41, 193, 194, 195
adrenaline *see* epinephrine
adrenergic receptors 195–198
adrenocorticosteroids *see* glucocorticoids
AGRP 209, 215

alkaline phosphatase 63, 136, 139, 142
allophenic mice 80
ampicillin 31
androgens 182, 183, 186–187, 188–189
angiotensin 179
angiotensinogen 179
anticodon 22
ap2 166, 168, 169
appetite 202, 204, 209, 210, 214
arachidonic acid 168, 176
arcuate (ARC) nucleus 96, 204, 208, 209, 214
ATP 63, 196
autocrine 37
autonomic nervous system (ANS) 192, 193
average daily gain 7

β-adrenergic receptors 196–198, 199, 200
β-agonists 42, 158, 196, 198, 199, 200
β-endorphins 215
beta oxidation 91–92, 167, 168
bHLH transcription factor 148, 149, 171
biglycan 62
biotechnology 27
blastocyst 55
body weight 2–3
bone 60, 61
bone canaliculi 64
bone lacuni 64
bone marrow 60, 64, 67
bone marrow stroma 133, 134, 142
bone matrix 61, 62, 65, 67
bone mineralization *see* ossification

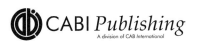
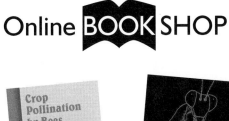

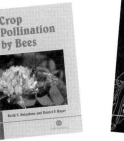
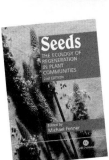
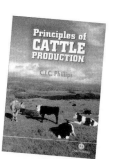